STONEY

The Waves And The Silver Lining

Published by MNJLS Books
First Edition
Also available in eBook ISBN: 978-0578-37181-8
Paperback ISBN: 978-0-578-37180-1

Dedication

This book is dedicated to Mark Stoneberg and all of those who helped in the search and support of our family.

ONE

"Turn it off! Turn it off! *"* My heart pounded at the muffled hair-raising sound from somewhere. *Was it outside? Inside?* I looked around puzzled. Then, the words became clearer and louder as heavy footsteps pounded through the house.

He now stood before me in the living room with one hand pointed to a speaker, his voice now in an unsteady, distressed whisper squeezing out his words, "Turn it off. Mom, *that's* what was playing in the background when you called to tell us dad went missing. I just can't listen to it anymore."

My mind whirled. It took several seconds for me to process what was happening.

It was my son, Lucas. I felt the pain in his eyes deep inside my belly—like a rabble of caged butterflies gone mad, confused and threatened in their surroundings, pushing and sparring against each other searching for an escape. Nothing like the fluttering you feel when watching a beautiful sunrise or smelling the first apple blossom in the spring. I moved slowly toward Lucas with my arms outstretched to hold him. I wanted to take the pain that I heard in his voice and saw in his eyes and move it far away. We stood hugging each other in the living room and sobbed as our torn hearts ripped further into unrecognizable fragments.

The song from my music playlist that our son Lucas had not heard since his dad's death was the somber song "Mad World" by Gary Jules. One of my favorite songs, but now with mixed emotions.

All around me are familiar faces, Worn out places, worn out faces
Bright and early for their daily races, Going nowhere, going nowhere
Their tears are filling up their glasses, No expression, no expression
Hide my head, I want to drown my sorrow
No tomorrow, no tomorrow…

Just minutes before Lucas had run frenzied into the living room upon my return home from Mexico one day earlier, I had clicked on my playlist after wrapping myself in a blanket and cradling into a stuffed chair next to the lit fireplace. The heat of the flames warmed my numb body and mind still engulfed in the surrealism of the previous excruciatingly painful nine days. It was the first day the four of us—me and my children—Jacob, Lucas, and Samantha were alone in our house where we had lived and loved as a family of five for so many years through the ups and downs, and trials and tribulations that life offers any one of us on this big blue planet of ours. We were two days away from Mark's funeral and I sat staring at the family photo of the five of us illuminated by the light in the wooden hutch, and I thought, *It was real. Why couldn't it be just a bad dream? We had so much more living to do as a couple and a family.* I hadn't slept or eaten much since his passing. *His passing.*

Now, we were suddenly a family of four with Mark ripped from our lives in a few horrific seconds. Or were we a family anymore? What were we without my husband and my children's father? A new normal? In my heart, mind, and soul, normal to me meant Mark and me and our three children. I have heard it said that the heart and mind are comprised in the soul, and that the soul defines the inner person—the culmination of all our knowledge and beliefs. All we had known was how to be a family of five. Where were we to go from here without our Mark?

TWO

Invitation to Sayulita

The planning for our vacation that ended in tragedy began on a crisp fall evening in 2012, when Mark and I met with friends, Kirk and his girlfriend Liz, at a local Minneapolis Mexican restaurant. Kirk had a special type of influence over Mark and could get him to try new things that he otherwise would have resisted. For instance, that night, the night that Mark and I drove to a Mexican restaurant several miles away in rush hour for a 5:30 dinner reservation in the middle of the week. Normally, Mark's lighthearted, yet emphatic, response would have been, "Hell no. I drive all day for work, I'm not going to drive anywhere in rush hour especially to a Mexican restaurant."

It was that time of day—rush hour. That time of year—chilly. That type of weather—rainy. And that kind of restaurant—Mexican. If it were any other person at any other time in our many years of marriage Mark never would have gone. But Kirk called him and the next thing I knew we were driving in traffic to a Mexican restaurant—and Mark didn't even like Mexican food. It was bizarre. I, on the other hand, like Mexican food and whenever Mark agreed to eat at a Mexican restaurant, he could always find a dish where he'd be able to re-create his own simple meal. He would order a chicken or beef dinner and then meticulously remove the smothering ingredients he called, *squigglies,* when referring to stir fried onions, peppers, and other vegetables, and push them off onto a different plate. With the exception for the need to cook certain vegetables such as potatoes, corn, or green beans, Mark preferred to eat raw vegetables. Another thing that would have bothered Mark about going to that particular restaurant is that there was no parking lot, only on-street parking, and we ended up parking two blocks away. Ordinarily, those combined circumstances would have made him want to stay home, but none of it bothered him a bit that night. Any other time his jaw clenching would have started and been seen visibly pulsating beneath his high cheek bones. He often clenched his jaw when he felt annoyed. But Kirk's request for Mark and me to join him and Liz for dinner that night seemed different than a typical spontaneous invitation.

As the four of us talked and ate—after Mark had successfully decontaminated his food of all squigglies—Kirk invited Mark and me to join him and Liz at his favorite remote haven in Sayulita, Mexico, for a time of relaxation and to learn how to surf. The trip was planned for February 2013, just five months away. Kirk knew that Mark and I were familiar with the culture in the area because we own a timeshare at a resort in Nuevo Vallarta, Mexico, about twenty miles south of Sayulita. But that is where the similarity ends. Kirk told us that Sayulita is a small, laid-back fishing and surf village with a population at the time of about 2,300 as compared to Nuevo Vallarta at over 125,000.

Kirk had been to Sayulita several times over the years as a single man to surf and stay on the beach in an extremely raw and rustic bungalow. In the late 1960's, it was "discovered" by surfers drawn there because of its consistent river mouth surf break making for great surfing, and described by many as the 'Crown Jewel' of the Riviera Nayarit. Kirk had often told Mark and me about his sacred getaway, but had never invited anyone, and certainly not a woman who might not feel safe in such primitive and sparse accommodations. He told us the only 'room' inside the bungalow was a bedroom with screenless window openings, and handmade bamboo shutters for privacy and protection from rainstorms. The rest of the bungalow consisted of a covered open area, with a kitchenette and small sitting area on a concrete floor that led to the white sand beach. It also had a covered open-air bathroom with six-foot bamboo walls for privacy. The unpurified running water was meant only for showering and handwashing. For drinking and dishwashing, it came equipped with a large freshwater container and attached hand pump.

Mark and I were enthusiastic and honored to have been invited knowing this was Kirk's personal paradise, and we had never surfed before. We were both strong swimmers and had body surfed over the years, but never on a surfboard. Kirk assured us that with several hours of practice and fortitude over a couple of days of falling fifty times or more off the surfboard, that we'd be hooked and want to advance to the next level. Over our years together, Mark and I had shared a deep sense of adventure and we became quickly intrigued with the idea of visiting Kirk's remote refuge. We said, "Yes," thinking it would be an exciting pre-retirement celebration. The four of us were destined for a spectacular time of fun in the sun in a small village on Mexico's Pacific coast.

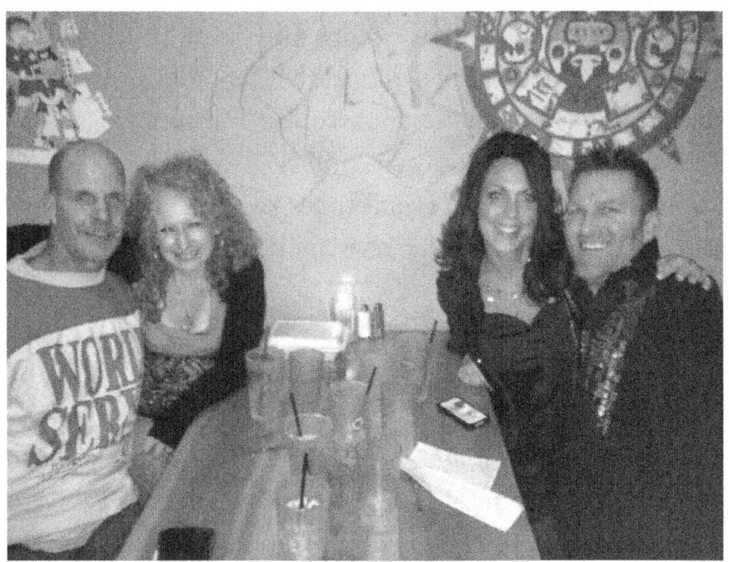

Mark, Me, Liz, and Kirk

When Kirk extended the invitation to us, Mark and I had been married for over twenty-six years, and Kirk and Liz had been dating for about two years.

Kirk and Liz met each other when Kirk was on a guy's golf weekend including Mark and other friends, and Liz was on a girl's weekend with her friends. As the story goes, the guys were at a bar hanging out when Liz and her girlfriends walked in. After a while Liz noticed Kirk looking at her and smiling from across the bar. So in a flirtatious move she walked over to Kirk, lightly flicked his hat, and kept walking. Before long, they were talking and out dancing with Mark agreeing to hold Liz's purse. When they came back from the dance floor Mark commented to Liz, "I can't believe you got Kirk out dancing. He doesn't dance." But Liz told Mark that Kirk had done the asking.

I met Liz for the first time a couple of months later in September of 2011, when Mark and I joined Kirk and her at an indoor simulated golf range, and again a month later at our twenty-fifth wedding anniversary party at one of our favorite local restaurants, Nona Rosa's. We sent out over two hundred invitations for our party, primarily inviting people to the reception thinking that the church ceremony to renew our vows would be a smaller family gathering, but we welcomed people to join us for the ceremony if they wished to do so. We assumed most people would have come only to the reception, but when we pulled into the church parking lot it was packed, and the church was filled as if it were a real wedding. It was a beautiful ceremony and a fantastic celebration afterward at the restaurant. The outpouring of love and support overwhelmed us.

It was great to see Liz again at our anniversary party and get to know her better. She and Kirk made a lovely couple; the synergy between the four of us was good as we shared the same interest in music, dancing, and golf. Liz lived about ninety miles away from Kirk where he lived in Minneapolis. Soon after he met Liz, Kirk traveled nearly every weekend to see her, and Mark told me he had never seen Kirk act like that before—so enamored with a woman to drive over an hour every weekend to be with her. Several months later, in 2012, Kirk asked Liz to move to Minneapolis to live with him, she accepted, and that's when the four of us started doing more things together.

Soon after the invitation from Kirk, we all started training. Mark and I started agility and strength training in our home gym—with heavy workout equipment—for the specific muscles and movement we would need for surfing. Kirk came over to work out with Mark a few times a week, and Liz and I trained separately on our own. There was one time, however, when I was training with Mark in our basement gym, and he wanted me to teach him the skill of hopping on a surfboard by doing some plyometric exercises—also called 'dynamic jump training.' Standing at 6'5", the first time Mark jumped up his head went right through the ceiling tile. Good thing it was a false ceiling and better yet that he did *not* hit a beam. Mark stood crunched over rubbing his head and looking up at the ceiling mumbling, "Well, I don't think we're going to do that again anytime soon."

I had been blessed to stay at home to raise all three children during their early years, while also making extra money training a few female clients in our home gym. When Jacob and Lucas were young and before Sami was born, I became a competitive body builder, and won championships in natural body building. At age thirty, after Sami was born, I took fifteen years off from competing. Then, at age forty-five I re-entered the competition, but the year before I re-entered, I wanted Sami to be on board with it, so I brought her to a contest so she could see what I would be doing. At age fifteen, she thought it was cool, so I trained for a year and participated in the master's division for women forty-five and over.

Mark worked out regularly as well over the years as we both knew the importance of staying fit at every age. Move ahead a couple of decades, and now Mark and I were going to learn to surf and continue fulfilling our already plentiful list of adventures we'd shared over our many years of marriage—with me in my late 40's and Mark in his late 50's. In addition to personal training, we watched and studied training videos about surfing.

We used a hard foam roller and practiced standing and shifting our weight to simulate the balance and motions required for surfing. I even had an opportunity to demonstrate this feat on a local daytime KSTP-TV show "Twin Cities Live" where I had become their "fitness guru" creating various workouts for their television audience.

Liz and I had gotten to know one another over the previous year and a half, but only as a foursome. As time moved closer to our trip to Sayulita, Mark and Kirk thought it would be good for Liz and me to visit our timeshare in Mexico as a great way for the two us to get to know each other better since we would be together for a week only three months away.

Liz and I thought it was a wonderful idea and were excited that it was only going to be the two of us, and it turned out to be a perfect week getting to know one another better starting with the airplane ride. We had tickets for coach, but when we got to the check-in, the ticket agent said for $99 she could upgrade us to first class. It was a big discount, so we jumped at the offer. As we sat in first class waiting for the other passengers to board, the flight attendant had served us bottomless glasses of mimosas. I sat with my back against the window with my legs propped up and cross-legged grilling Liz as I wanted to know everything about her. Four hours flew by and before we knew it, we landed in Puerto Vallarta. Everything moved effortlessly from our time on the airplane, to having our suitcases waiting for us on the carousel, to quickly catching a twenty-minute shuttle ride straight to the resort in Nuevo Vallarta.

The resort sits at the end of a peninsula and our suite has breathtaking views of the ocean and surrounding palm trees. Our time getting to know one another was easy and natural. We relaxed, walked the beach, talked a lot, ate, and simply enjoyed the rich local culture.

We happened to be in Mexico on December 12th, 2012, and we whimsically wrote 12/12/12, in the sand that day on the beach. We learned about each other's upbringing with me growing up in a closely knit family in a small town, and that Liz's life was also closely knit on a large family farm. I developed a high level of respect for her learning how she and her siblings and parents raised crops and built silos together.

Upon our return home, Mark and Kirk were happy to know that Liz and I got along so well. Shortly after that, with retirement approaching soon for Mark, along with the guys' love of golf, the four of us hired a realtor to find side-by-side townhomes on a golf course in Arizona to escape the cold Minnesota winters.

A couple of weeks after our girl's excursion to Mexico, and two months away from our Sayulita trip, Mark and I had a small New Year's Eve party at our house that included Kirk, Liz, our brother-in-law Brian, and our friend Brian (Bubba). Over the years Mark and I had hosted large New Year's Eve parties in our home which included family, friends, and our children's friends. The parties were always wonderful, yet so big and so busy that Mark and I never really got to take it all in, or even talk to each other until after everyone left and we went to bed.

But December 31st, 2012, was different with just the six of us. We managed to include a bit of physical fitness into our festivities, and started out the night by going downstairs to the gym and having silly contests like who could stand on the foam roller the longest, how many pull ups could we do, and other agility movements for surfing and other things like the hiking we'd be doing in Sayulita. That is how excited we were for the vacation just a few weeks away.

The six of us then moved to the family room and played simple little card games and had a marvelous, low-key evening with lots of laughs and joking around. That New Year's Eve—which would be our last one together—was one of the most intimate times Mark and I had spent bringing in the new year.

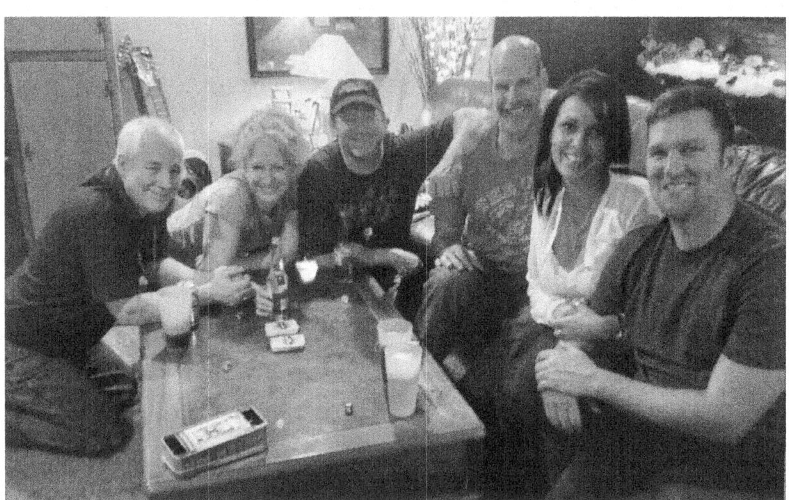

Brian, Me, Bubba, Mark, Liz, and Kirk

THREE

Stoney

To others, I lovingly referred to Mark as *my* Mark. Most of his friends and all of his co-workers called him Stoney, short for Stoneberg, except for Kirk, who called him Old Sac. And others, primarily family members, often referred to Mark and me together as 'big Mark and Nancy', not only regarding Mark's height of 6'5" and weight of 220 pounds versus my shortness of 5'1½" and 110 pounds, but also to distinguish between my brother, Mark, and his wife, Nancy. Mark's big stature and my tininess seemed always a big deal to him. He loved that I was so small and that he could easily pick me up and frolic around.

Mark was an intelligent and witty man who embraced meaningful conversations. He lived his Christian faith, not with words, but in attitude and actions. He was friendly and engaging with others but remained reserved about fully revealing himself too quickly. Upon first meeting Mark, some found his sizeable, physically fit stature, and deep-set blue eyes, that seemed to look right through you, a little bit intimidating. However, the instant he flashed his broad smile revealing his gorgeous white teeth, and through his deep buttery voice flowed kind and clever words, people realized he was a softie inside. He had a grateful heart and caring attitude toward others, especially toward his family and close buddies. Mark loved deeply. He had a type of open unreserved love for people, and he wasn't the kind of guy to say, *Hey, love ya man!* He would never toss that word around lightly. He was a man waiting for the next challenge. If anyone told him he could not do something, he set out to prove them wrong. Not in an arrogant manner, but he loved a challenge. He was extremely motivated in all aspects of his life, and if he said he was going to do something—he did it.

Mark had a rock-solid memory about dates and times from years ago, and a knack for trivia leaving people astonished at what he knew. He was focused and had a strong analytical mind. Math came naturally to him, and he liked working with his hands. That is why he excelled at his job as a high-voltage electrical lineman at Xcel Energy. He easily understood the complicated math involved in the study of electricity, and chose a career that allowed him to use both his mechanical and physical abilities. The job was an excellent fit for his adrenaline-seeking personality and is ranked one of the fifteenth most dangerous jobs in America. He worked around live wires and circuitry with some jobs requiring him to climb wooden poles strapped with heavy tools, and sometimes hiking up sixty-foot poles in areas inaccessible for his bucket truck. He worked in every type of weather and knew that safety procedures were of utmost importance. And he brought a similar kind of focus, analysis, thrill-seeking, and safeguarding inherent in his workday world into our family life and his friendships as well. He was a brave man surrounded by danger every day. He often told me, "You know, my job is plenty safe…as long as I don't make *one* mistake."

Mark and I had traveled consistently throughout our marriage with at least one vacation per year specifically with just the two of us. It could mean getting in the car in the springtime and heading to some warmer states. In the earlier years we drove his 1977 black 2-door Lincoln Mark V that he had scrimped and saved to buy used in 1983. It didn't matter where we went or how far. We just drove and traveled together. We'd stop at various landmarks along the way, and play a round of golf at public courses here and there. It was important to Mark that we did that. In fact, it was at one of my wedding showers in which everyone wrote down a bit of advice to the bride, that his mother lovingly wrote, "Don't ever forget who came first." Meaning, keep your relationship strong and vital so you continue growing closer to each other. It was a lot of work for me to prepare for the trips with organizing our children's activities, but it was important for him that we take time for just the two of us, and I was completely on board. My folks would come to town from Grand Forks, North Dakota, to stay with the children, and the two of us would head out for a week or so.

We also took family vacations with our children in the earlier years visiting one of Minnesota's 10,000 lakes and renting a cabin during the summer, or going home to visit my family in North Dakota. I often refer to our children with the same term of endearment as to how I reference *my* Mark, not simply by mentioning their names, but as *my* Jacob, *my* Lucas, *my* Samantha, aka Jake, Luke, and Sami.

When Mark and I traveled together with friends to warm places in the winter, it was often with a group of people on our volleyball teams. Some on Mark's men's team, some from our coed team. We had lots of fun together and often took on the resort staff or locals on the beach in a game of volleyball. But never would we go anywhere on Mark's mom's birthday in January which was prime time for winter vacations. One time our volleyball group planned a vacation where we would've been gone on her birthday, and Mark said, "Well, I hope you all have a great time. I won't be gone on my mom's birthday." So, they changed the date.

As time moved on, Mark enjoyed playing on softball teams with our sons Jacob and Lucas. Though softball and volleyball had been Mark's primary sports interests, he suffered with various aches and pains, and with retirement approaching he felt that golf would be a good way to continue staying active and in shape, and something we could do together.

In 2011, we met with our financial advisor, Jeff, and he showed Mark that he was in a great position to move forward and enjoy early retirement at age fifty-nine just two years away in June 2013. Mark responded to Jeff, "Does that mean I don't always have to use coupons to golf?"

Mark was so ready for retirement as there were structural changes beginning to happen at Xcel Energy, and the timing was right for him to be done, and for us to start our new chapter in life together. He planned to keep working part-time as a contractor in the electrical energy industry in a capacity other than as a lineman, and the part-time work would provide him with a sense of purpose and structure he had been used to for so many years, while still leaving much time for family, sports, and other interests.

FOUR

The Night Before Going To Sayulita

Move ahead to our vacation to Sayulita, with Jacob now twenty-five, Lucas twenty-three, and Sami eighteen and in high school. Jacob owned his own home nearby, and Lucas and Sami lived at home and were gone a lot either working or just doing their own thing.

Now that they were older, when Mark and I went on vacations, we simply reminded them that we were leaving town the next day. One of them was always in charge of the house, and Jacob would drop in often when we were gone. We always wondered if there might be a party, but they were good about that and always used good judgement. We wouldn't necessarily see them before we left, but would let them know where we were staying and that we'd see them in a week.

However, the night before the vacation to Sayulita an unusual situation happened. Our nephew Trevor, Mark's brother Michael's son, was soon deploying with the National Guard to Afghanistan. Trevor planned to have a Friday night party for his guy friends and another party on Saturday night for the family. We told Trevor we were leaving on Saturday and asked if we could come to the Friday night party. "Of course, cool," he said.

We then called Jacob, Lucas, and Sami and they were all able to make it. Mark and I were happy that all five of us would be there because getting all of us together had become more difficult over the years considering everyone's schedules, and it was the first time since the children were young that all of us would be together the night before we left on our vacation. It turned out to be a magical time together.

The party was held at an entertainment restaurant filled with arcade games, bowling lanes, and billiard tables. After we spent some quality time with Trevor and Mark's brothers and other people we knew at his 'guys' party, Mark, Jacob, Lucas, Sami, and I hung together in a pack the rest of the evening. We shot pool and played games as a five-some the rest of the night. It was a blast—one of those great, great nights with lots of fun and joking around.

Jacob and Lucas had driven to the party together, and when it ended, we hugged them both and said good night, and to Lucas we said our usual, "Love you, see you in a week," as we would be seeing Jacob the next morning for our ride to the airport. Then Mark and I drove Sami to a girlfriend's house to spend the night, and again we hugged, said we loved one another, and that we would see her in a week.

FIVE

Vacation Day 1—Saturday, February 23rd

Early the next morning, Jacob drove Mark, me, Kirk, and Liz to the airport. Mark and I hugged Jacob, and said our usual, "We love you! See you in a week!" And off we went into the terminal.

No one could have known those hugs and words, *I love you, see you in a week,* would be the final tender sentiments shared between a loving father and his precious children.

We packed two big bags for the week. With Mark's concerns about being in a small village and wanting his food simple and without squigglies, we strategically packed one suitcase filled with food that he liked, along with a box of wine—for gosh sakes—for me. Why we thought that Sayulita wouldn't have any wine or food we liked, I don't know, but we ended up having two giant suitcases one of which was filled completely with perishables, the other with clothing. We froze all the food inside baggies and ensured the suitcase weighed just under fifty pounds so we wouldn't have to pay the extra fee. Mark and I never considered that we should or should not bring a suitcase filled with food—we were bringing it anyway.

All the bags checked in fine at the Minneapolis/St. Paul International Airport, and we settled in at a bar sipping our early morning cocktails and eating breakfast while waiting for the flight.

A short while later we boarded the airplane. Kirk had booked the flight for all of us, and he intentionally booked the emergency exit seats to surprise Mark out of consideration for his height so he'd have substantially more leg room than in a regular coach seat, and for himself as well, as he too stood over six feet tall. Mark didn't like flying even in the best seat with ample leg room because it was just too cramped. And of course, there was more than enough leg room for me and my smaller frame.

The four of us sat across the aisle from each other. Normally, Mark and I would converse with the friends we traveled with, but this time it was unusually different. Mark and I talked only with each other, and I believe fate likely had some part in that. We discussed things we had never talked about. Ironically, we talked about things like who of the children would be the executor of the estate in the event of our deaths. Things that were really deep and very sad yet lots of fun conversation too—*hours* of passionate deliberation.

About two hours into the flight, during a short intermission from our playful and heavy conversations, the flight attendant handed us custom forms and I told Mark I'd fill them out. When it came to the question asking if we were declaring any food items, we'd never had to think about that in previous travels as we just had little snicky snacks in our carry-on bags. I leaned over Mark and across the aisle to Kirk and asked, "What should I write down about the food in the suitcase?" He looked at me with big eyes, shaking his head no, his index finger to his lips mouthing *shhhhh,* as if saying, *stop, be quiet, don't say anymore.* Mark didn't pick up on any of it. I was confused about Kirk's cautioning me, but I certainly understood what *shhhhh* meant and understood he was saying don't talk about it and don't write it down. So I took his advice and didn't write anything down, and the flight continued with Mark and I back in our own world of talking about anything and everything—our hearts and minds entwined like never before.

We landed around 10 am in Puerto Vallarta so we still had a lot of daytime ahead of us for fun. Inside the terminal, as we walked toward the baggage claim, Kirk asked us, "What was going on with you two on the airplane? You acted like newlyweds starting a new life together. What were you talking about?"

Mark turned to Kirk, clenched his jaw, and said, "What's your point?" We all laughed. That was Mark's playful classic response to avoid answering a question. And I get it. Our time on the airplane was unusual and it was beautiful because we truly did talk about so many things that we hadn't talked about for years—or ever.

Mark and I looked at each other, and I responded, "It was about everything—happy things, sad things, it was about death and dying and life and living. It was about Mark's upcoming retirement in four months on his fifty-ninth birthday, and to celebrate his forty years at Xcel Energy. We discussed plans to take dance lessons, and to find a transition counselor to learn how to move forward together as empty nesters, while still spending time with our children; and how we looked forward to a winter place in Arizona with you and Liz where our children, and other family and friends could visit, and we touched base on many other travel plans and dreams. And…I don't know where the time went, but it sure was fun!"

We claimed our luggage and Kirk took me aside smiling mischievously, and whispered, "Give the suitcase with the food in it to Old Sac."

I looked at him confused. He motioned for me to slide the food suitcase over to Mark.

Mark had no idea that Kirk told me not to declare the food. And the reason Kirk told me to give it to Mark is that if we got stopped by Mexican customs, and if there was going to be legal action with someone getting arrested, that Mark would do better in jail than me with Mark standing fearlessly strong and tall, and me strong also yet over a foot shorter. So here I was after an amazing flight of passionately connecting with my husband, and I slid the bag over to him setting him up for a fall. I looked at Kirk and Liz, shaking my head, softly giggling, and thinking, *Oh my god…this is crazy.*

We all stood together waiting for each of our bags to get the green light for "go" or red light for "stop" for a bag check. My palms were sweating as I looked alternately at Mark in front of me totally oblivious as to what could happen in the next few seconds, and behind me at Kirk and Liz, mouthing, *Oh my god.*

Well, we made it through. All our bags got the green light. The moment we got through the customs gate, Mark stopped, opened the food suitcase, and grabbed a sandwich. Kirk, Liz, and I stood looking at him laughing.

"What?" he said, eyeing us with suspicion.

We told him what happened with me sliding the suitcase over to him, and in his deep belly laugh, he agreed with us saying, "Yeah, I would've done better in jail than you with your height and curly red hair and freckles." Then he looked down at his sandwich, lifted it up offering a toast, and took a bite.

We walked outside the airport and saw a man standing in front of us holding a sign with Kirk's last name written on it. The man holding the sign was our own private shuttle bus driver there to whisk us away to Sayulita. Mark and I were both wowed by the gesture from Kirk and Liz. Mark turned to them with eyes tearing, his head bowed to them saying, "I've never had anything like this done for me."

Neither had I, and I was blown away as well, but Mark's feelings of appreciation deeply penetrated his soul because of his good friend's kindness to privately transport us to his paradise. Mark and I hadn't thought about how we'd get to the village, probably by bus, but we were definitely not expecting a private shuttle ride.

The first and only stop on the shuttle was to get beer for the hour-long ride to Sayulita. We settled in and Liz said, "Let's take a selfie of the four of us!"

Selfies were a fairly new thing back in 2013 and I personally had never taken one before that day, so we gathered together and I snapped the first photo on our trip, all of us whooping it up on the shuttle with none of us knowing it would be the last one of the four of us. And Mark's smile in that photo, oh my goodness, he was so, so happy—almost glowing.

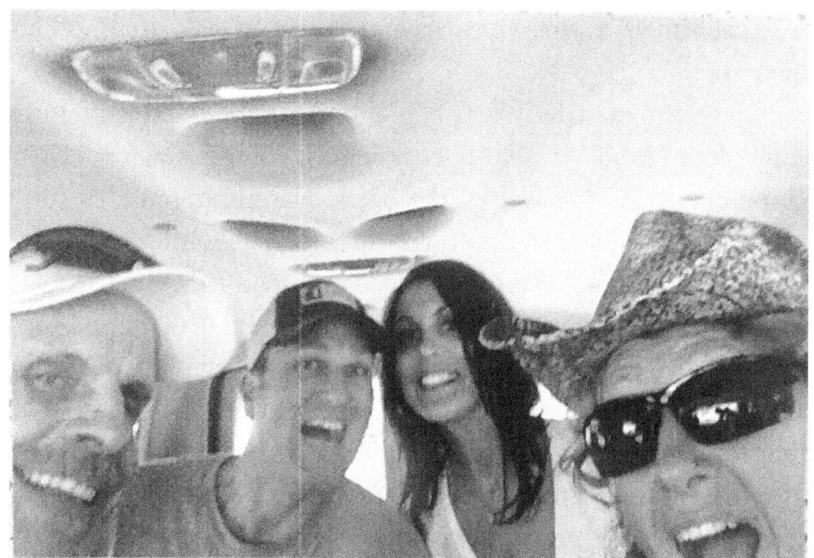

Mark, Kirk, Liz, and Me

Once past the big city limits, we wound through the mountains on a shoulderless narrow two-lane road beautifully framed on both sides with thickly forested lush green plants, palm trees, and other trees that overarched the roadway creating tree tunnels. Small thatched roofed and tin roofed open shelters dotted the route providing travelers a place to rest and buy local wares and food including fresh fruit, cold coconut, homemade bread, and *dulces regionales* which is Spanish for regional candies. Oh, so delicioso.

When we turned off the main road into the village of Sayulita with its cobblestone dirt roads, the inviting sound of Mariachi music in the air, and vibrantly colored restaurants and shops, we *knew* our vacation was going to be something incredibly special.

The driver asked Kirk where we were staying.

Kirk responded, "The trailer park."

Mark and I looked at each other quizzically, *trailer park?* Well, it turns out that the trailer park is where the bungalows are located and where many snowbirds keep their campers year-round, and so it had become known as the trailer park.

The driver dropped us off, we grabbed our bags and dragged them across the deep sand to the ocean-side of our bungalow where the intoxicating enormous expanse of the ocean warmly greeted us fifty yards away. We had been teleported into an old-world tranquil, picturesque, and inspiring tropical utopia. We experienced the kind of peace that instantly engulfs and relaxes the body with the feel and smell of the warm balmy ocean breeze, and the concert of tropical birds serenading all around us. Kirk had been right about his humbly unique sacred getaway. The two-story bungalow looked and felt exotic and ruggedly comfortable. Mark and I stayed on the lower level with Kirk and Liz in the loft above. Just like Kirk had told us, the entire area was open-air under one roof with a bedroom, kitchen, living room, and bathroom. The concrete floor extended out to the white sand beach with the ocean essentially at our doorstep. We noticed the large container of drinkable water that Kirk had told us about with a hand pump that we had to strong arm down, unlike big water coolers at home where a press of a button or flip of a lever would produce a steady flow. We pushed open old weatherworn French doors leading to the bedroom which was the only semi-secure area on our level. Semi-secure because just a slight push on the doors popped them right open.

Mark and I looked at each other smiling, *Ok this is cool, quaint, sexy…unusually romantic.* We now understood what Kirk had told us the year before when he described how rustic it was…and we were thrilled to be there.

Right away, the biggest concern for Mark was how to lock up our stuff—money, phones, jewelry—as we were going to be gone surfing and doing other things during the day. The stairway to Kirk and Liz's level above had a gated locked door so they had some security, and we figured they'd let us keep our valuables up there, but instead of bothering them with that, Mark got creative. While we unpacked, I noticed Mark looking high and low and climbing around the bedroom, and I chuckled trying to figure out what the heck he was doing. We brought a lot of cash, and he was searching for places to hide it.

In retrospect it was a good thing that I was in the room. Had I not been in there watching him putting a little roll of money here, and a roll of money there all around the room, I wouldn't have known where any of it was for what was ahead down the line.

We finished unpacking our things around noon and Kirk wanted to surf right away. Though Mark, Liz, and I had been readying our bodies to surf, we had never surfed before and knew we'd be doing a lot of it in the coming days, so the three of us chose to hang on the beach and watch Kirk show us the ropes.

While Mark and I waited for Kirk and Liz to come down to the main level of the bungalow, Mark sat on the steps taking in the sights. As Kirk and Liz walked down the steps, we all heard Mark shout out in his deep voice, "Nancy Elizabeth! Nancy Elizabeth! There's bananas in that tree!" It was so funny. He had never seen a real live banana tree and neither had I. So many things about our trip to that point had been new and exhilarating and we were loving everything about it. Mark's endearing term for me was often my first and middle name, Nancy Elizabeth, and besides calling him *my* Mark when speaking about him to others—I called him sweetheart.

The four of us walked down the beach to the surf school so Kirk could rent a surfboard. I wore a sundress and carried my sandals. The sand was a welcomed foot massage—my toes wriggled free from the confines of my winter boots left behind at home in the frozen tundra. White snow to white sand: a lovely transition. Wispy clouds floated softly across the sky. Jewel-blue waves rippled gently. We watched sea gulls squawking, flying, and dive-bombing for food with a variety of other birds scampering on the beach. The air was thick with the smell of the ocean, the cheerful sound of a nearby steel drum, and the tease of spicy aromas from restaurants along the beach front.

With Kirk in the water on his board, Liz, Mark, and I settled on the sand in front of the row of beachside restaurants and watched him effortlessly ride the waves. He made it look easy and the three of us wondered if we'd be able to surf half as good as him during our weeklong vacation, because we had also watched beginner surfers near him pop up on a board only to quickly fall back into the water.

A beach vendor approached us displaying a wonderful presentation of precious stones and medallions resting on a black velvet clothe. He spoke broken English and situated himself next to us. He picked up a stone and wrapped it beautifully in silver wire creating a unique pendant in just a few short minutes. We looked on fascinated with his artistry and skill. In all of our previous travels, never had we been approached by a jeweler making beautiful pendants right on the spot.

Mark turned to me and asked if I would like one.

"Oh my gosh, yes!"

I picked out a rich golden amber stone. The jeweler asked Mark if he wanted to help, and he jumped right in. It was so cool. The two of them cradled the stone in a small shell and together they wrapped it and attached it to an adjustable leather cord. Mark was so excited and asked if I wanted another one. I did, and I picked out a black Indianhead medallion and Mark and the jeweler creatively wrapped the wire around that one too. Mark was having the time of his life.

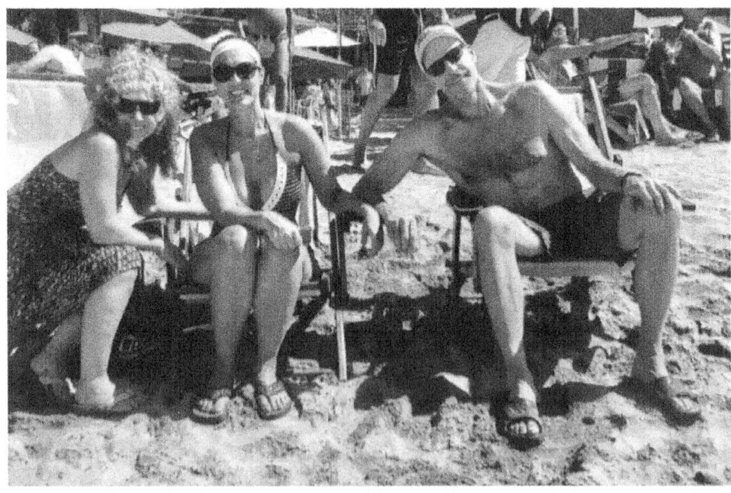

Me, Liz, and Mark

After Kirk got his surfing fix, he joined us on the beach and a short while later the four of us strolled the quarter mile back to the bungalow, changed clothes, and then walked back down the same beach a quarter mile to the village to eat dinner at one of several restaurants.

I changed into a little hippie outfit with a cool fringed purse slung across my body. I thought it would be fun to listen to the songs I had created on a playlist as we walked, so I placed my small battery-operated speakers inside my purse. They were a little heavy and the wires a bit cumbersome, but it worked. As we walked along the beach, we experienced the neatest and funniest thing. People of all ages followed us— commenting, laughing, and dancing to the music coming from my purse. What a fabulous time the four of us had walking and listening to our favorite music playing in my purse with a parade of folks dancing behind us.

In planning our vacation my only responsibility was to create a music playlist, which was unusual for me as I was the one, on all our previous vacations, who took care of most, if not all, of the planning. But all anyone cared about on this vacation was that I create a playlist that represented all four of us. So I did. I created a list with over two hundred songs. Initially, I thought I'd have about a hundred songs, but that didn't happen because I had so many ideas about Kirk who enjoyed his type of pop music, Liz who loved country music, along with my eclectic interests, so I grabbed songs left and right off of Pandora for the three of us, but for Mark I did something different.

Over the fall and winter months before our trip, Mark and I sat in the family room together. While Mark watched TV on the weekends, I played songs on Pandora. His only job was to give me a thumbs up or a thumbs down, and if it was a thumbs up, I bought the song. That's how I was able to have so many songs that truly represented Mark, and those sessions with him had been so precious. Apparently, I nailed it because Mark, Kirk, and Liz completely enjoyed the songs.

The sights, sounds, smells, and colors of the town awed both Mark and I, as we'd never embraced local culture at that level. Mark seemed entranced. He sauntered silently down the cobblestone walkway wearing a pleasant grin while absorbing our festive surroundings.

Mark had recently gotten the green light from his doctor that all was fine with him after receiving results from a series of exams—some general, others specific—and that he was a healthy and strong fifty-eight-year-old man. He had struggled his entire life with chronic back pain, as he was born with a touch of scoliosis which made him stand and walk a little crooked when he was tired. He also lived with pain in his neck, shoulder, elbow, and knees from working as a lineman and being an avid athlete. Mark and I would joke around with each other personifying the poor ibuprofen that he had to take as it wondered where to start first in his body as if saying, *What do you want me to do in here? It's all inflamed! Where am I to go first?*

A few months before our vacation, Mark had undergone a long-awaited right knee replacement. The doctors thought he would need both knees replaced, but because of a successful rehabilitation with the right knee, it took pressure off the left, and he didn't need the left one replaced after all. The main reason Mark waited so long for the replacement is that his doctors had told him after the procedure that he wouldn't be able to run again. However, a friend of his had undergone the same surgery, and after a full rehabilitation with a new knee, he was able to run and play softball again. When Mark heard that, he felt that if his friend could recover then he certainly could too. It was part of his personality to love the challenge, so, Mark moved ahead with the surgery and fully recovered, and just like his friend, he was able to run and play softball.

Amazingly, his other pains subsided along the way as well. Maybe because he was living on the verge of retirement. Who knows? But it was the most pain-free he had been in his life, and the man was going to learn to surf because he felt so terrific.

As the four of us moved through the village market, Liz and I occasionally dashed over to various shops to ogle the jewelry, hats, and clothing, and then hurried off to catch up with Mark and Kirk. We basked in the welcoming yellows, reds, purples, blues, and greens emblazoned on the buildings, in the artwork for sale, and on the rows upon rows of symbolic multi-colored Mexican flags strung above each street blowing gently in the warm breeze. As we walked around the village looking for a place to eat dinner, I will never forget turning down one of the streets in the Sayulita Town Square and seeing an amazing scene right out of a storybook. Directly in front of us stood a three-story skinny, skinny building with long thatched roofing and potted plants hanging from each level with open decks on all three levels. My heart skipped a beat. I stopped, pointed, and said to Mark, "That, *that* building, if it's a restaurant can we eat there?"

Mark sounded so sweet saying, "Of course we can Nancy Elizabeth, whatever you want."

Sure enough, it was a restaurant. We went in and asked to sit on the top floor balcony where we enjoyed breathtaking views for our first meal in Sayulita. I ordered an amazingly delicious pineapple generously filled with shrimp, and Mark, he was able to order a dish without squigglies in it, and Kirk and Liz ordered their favorite dishes as well. The trip started out so perfectly—the airplane ride, a private shuttle, a first-ever selfie, rustic bungalow, sitting on the beach, Kirk surfing, Mark making jewelry, walking along the multi-colored village streets in the warm tropical breeze, and enjoying a fabulous dinner with our good friends as we watched the sunset from the enchanted restaurant balcony—all of it felt so magnificent.

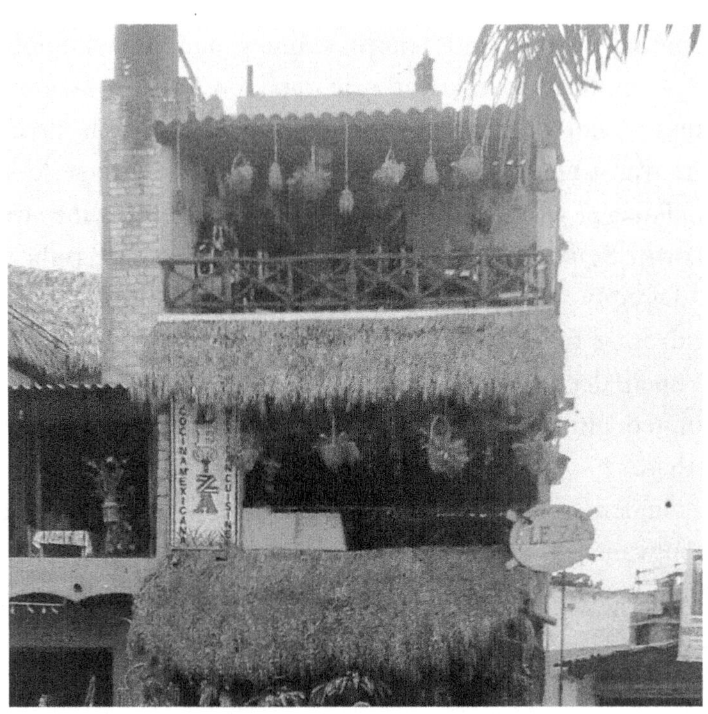

Skinny Restaurant Building

Dusk settled in as the four of us wandered back to the bungalow to relax the rest of the evening. It's easy to walk almost anywhere in Sayulita and nearly impossible to get lost. There's only one road in and one road out with no stop lights or stop signs. As we walked, Mark noticed a man and a young boy across the street standing next to a pick-up truck with its bed filled with baked goods. Mark pointed and said, "Let's go over there."

I looked at him perplexed. Mark didn't eat sweets. He was extremely health conscious. We walked to the rear of the bakery truck displaying a beautiful arrangement of freshly made cookies, bars, donuts, and cakes. It was a man and his son who owned the bakery. Mark chuckled as he pointed to different selections, like a kid in a candy store, as the boy placed the goodies in small paper bags, each holding only a few pieces. He bought dozens. I watched Mark in amazement knowing the only reason he was buying the sweets was to support the man and his son. I knew darn well he wasn't going to eat any of it. It was fun to see him so whimsical as that was unlike his more practical nature. Yes, he was a loving and giving man, but I'd never seen him so mischievously impulsive before.

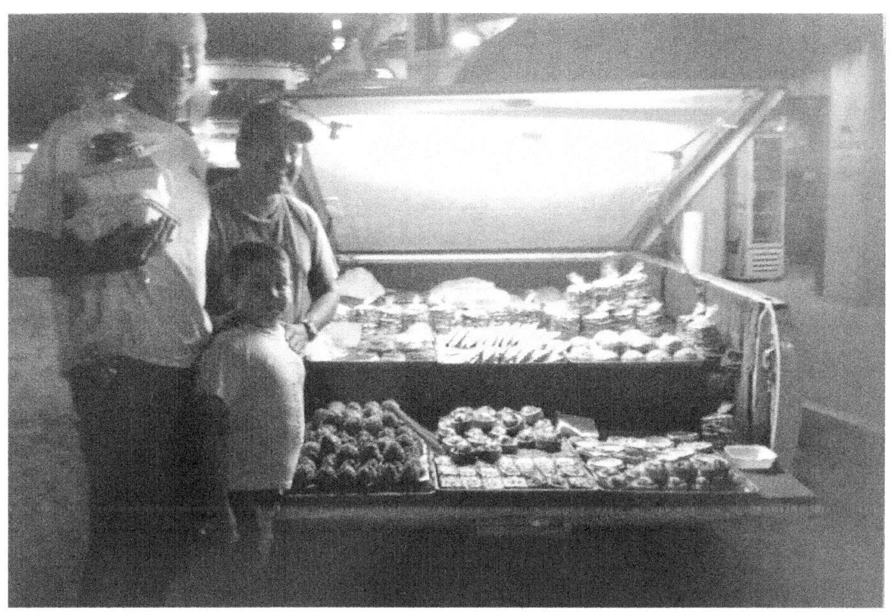
Mark with baker and baker's son

We continued our several block walk back to the bungalow laughing and balancing our overloaded arms with the restaurant leftovers and several bags of treats. The four of us relished the rest of the evening gazing out at the nearly full moonlit ocean while chatting and enjoying the music on our playlist.

SIX

Vacation Day 2—Sunday, February 24th

The next morning, we woke up fresh anticipating our first day of surfing. Mark commented to me about what a great night's sleep he had. I don't remember him ever saying that before. Normally, he had to sleep flat on his back to help ease his back pain, and while attempting to stay in one position all night, he would prop pillows on both sides of his head, cinch a beach towel tightly around his waist for support, and place more pillows under his knees, but eventually he ended up tossing, turning, and repositioning all night still waking up with a painful back. It must have been the fresh ocean air and the sounds of the waves that lulled him to sleep and kept him asleep. I was so happy for him. Both Kirk and Mark were beyond excited for our first day of surfing, but Liz and I were super nervous. We were excited but anxious at the same time as we didn't know what to fully expect; assuming we'd be floundering like the beginner surfers we saw the day before when we watched Kirk surf.

So, here we were ready to put our months of skills training to the test. We walked a quarter mile to the surf school on the southside of the beach known as 'the sandbar.'

Before entering the water, the surf school provides a mandatory half-hour land instruction about equipment, safety, and technique followed by one hour of surf instruction in the water.

We repeatedly practiced the following steps on our surfboards on the sand. We first learned how to lay on the board with our body centered and toes touching the back (tail), and how to pop up on the board by first placing our hands flat on the board, not on the sides (rails), next to our chest. Next step, a pushup with toes tucked on the tail of the surfboard without knees, waist, and legs touching the board. Then slide the back foot forward on the board keeping it bent, and quickly slide the front foot forward standing with knees bent and arms out for balance always looking forward and not down.

They taught us about two techniques—the 'punch through' and the 'turtle roll' in order to get beyond the white-water waves, and not get pushed back to shore. We learned how to carry the board by the front (nose) close and perpendicular to our side and walk to chest high water before getting on the board. They told us to paddle hard and fast on our belly with forearms deep and perpendicular to the board, as more speed equals more control, and about six feet before reaching the oncoming white-water to 'punch through' by grabbing the rails, push down on the board with chest up, and hold on tightly until the white-water passes between our body and the board. The 'turtle roll' was used to get past bigger white-water waves and not get pushed back, which means at about six feet before the white-water reaches you, take a deep breath, grab the rails besides your chest and turn yourself and the board upside down in the water, wait a few short seconds for the wave to pass over, then flip back over by pulling on one rail and pushing on the other while kicking to get back up.

By the end of the beach training, Mark, Liz, and I felt like we had a good handle on how to get past the white-water and pop up on the board and were excited to get out there and try it. We then followed the instructors into the water for further training.

Easy enough, right? Oh my gosh. Learning about the techniques on the sand made it seem easy, but sand doesn't move. Once you're out in the water, just getting on the board and staying on it is tough, much less trying to get beyond the white-water waves to pop up on the board. We fell off the board before we even got fully onto it. And every time we fell off the board, guess what? The tide brought us back in and we had to paddle back out to try to get beyond the white-water. The amount of work it took to paddle back out just to have a wave bring us back in was ridiculous. Thank goodness for the board leash around our ankles preventing our boards from floating away after a wipeout or injuring another surfer. And fortunately, Liz and I wore swim shorts and a long tank top acting as a rash guard, because our skin got really scratched up wrestling with the surfboards—and the surfboards always won.

In the beach training we learned about common mistakes for beginner surfers, and I know I made every one of them. When I mastered getting on and staying on the board on my belly, and then tried to 'punch through' the white water, I found I wasn't paddling with enough speed to push through the wave. I was physically fit from head to toe with a good sense of balance and strong arms for paddling, but those waves challenged every ounce of my strength. I also found I wasn't staying exactly perpendicular to the wave. How could I with the waves pushing the board sideways with me ending up at an angle and getting pushed back or flipping over? When I tried to use the 'turtle roll,' I again found myself not perpendicular to the wave or the surfboard nose wasn't underwater, and I got pushed back. Or if I turned upside down too soon or too late and wasn't perpendicular to the waves, I got pushed back. My skin had taken a beating with rashes and bruises forming on my arms and legs from so much contact with the board.

Mark, Liz, and I spent an hour in the water, up and down; up and down, trying our hardest to stay on the board while Kirk surfed effortlessly nearby. The three of us were exhausted. After a while I thought, *I don't want to do this anymore. I just want to sit here on my board.* And I wondered if I was ever going to get up on the board and feel a wave beneath me. But Kirk was a pro. He made it look so easy. He encouraged us saying he thought we did well for our first day, and said tomorrow would be a better day now that we had the basics down. He also said the waves were rougher than usual in the area especially for beginners. The instructors told us the same thing. We called it quits after the hour of toppling in the waves—the score 0 to 1 with the waves in first place.

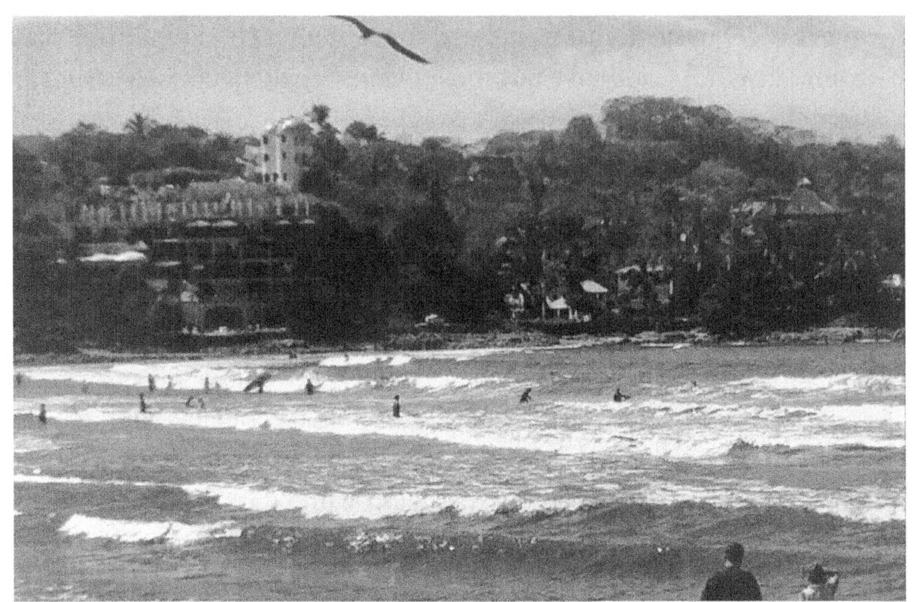

Waves on Sayulita's south side of beach

We limped across the sand to put our boards away and wobbled to the bungalow to rest and change clothes before walking into the village to experience *Sayulita Days*. Kirk told us about the annual weeklong celebration happening in the village with carnival rides, games, rodeos, food booths, and art and clothing kiosks.

Sunday includes all of the activities of the week, but adds a morning parade to include numerous marching bands comprised of school-age children dressed brightly and impeccably in their uniforms. The entire town shows up for the parade and to delight in the horsemen dressed in fancy cowboy attire with their dancing horses in the town square. Upon our arrival, every restaurant and every inch of outside space overflowed with people. We situated ourselves on a restaurant balcony to take in the merriment around us. The four of us ordered margaritas. When the waitress brought the drinks to our table, she placed two strawberry blended margaritas in front of Liz and me, and the regular margaritas on the rocks in front of Mark and Kirk. But our orders had been exactly the opposite.

When we switched around the drinks, the waitress looked puzzled at the two six-foot-tall-plus muscular men in tank tops as she pointed to the fruity slushy drinks in front of them, and then laughed that it was the women who had ordered theirs on the rocks. It *was* quite funny.

We had a perfect view of the parade from the balcony and of the numerous bands dotted around the grounds playing lively traditional music with horns, drums, and guitars generating a cheerful, invigorating energy. We watched men blow fire from their mouths, and horsemen waiting their turn to enter the circle of surrounding people to display their talent of horse dancing. We'd never heard of or seen anything like dancing horses before. One by one, the cowboys rode in on their well-groomed horses, positioned themselves in front of one of the bands, and proceeded to dance in step to the rhythm of the music.

At one point, Mark turned to me and said, "Nancy Elizabeth you have to take a video to show the kids!" I couldn't get my phone on video mode fast enough. It was extraordinary.

Sometimes there were two or three horses in the ring dancing, like a dance off, with riders on their backs moving in perfect unison together. Each rider sat tall and proud in the saddle leading his horse to move all four legs to prance delicately in place, and then step several feet sideways in one direction, twirl around, and then step back the other way. The horses went down on their bellies. They bent down on their knees. And they bowed to the audience. It was a show of amazing beauty and grace. And it was a competition that was scheduled to go on for hours. The four of us watched and cheered for well over an hour, and then decided to walk to eat dinner at a restaurant that Kirk claimed made the best fish tacos in town.

We made our way through the dense crowd inside the restaurant and out onto the dusty village street. As we left the area, Mark somehow spotted two evil-looking dogs on top of a flat-roofed short building intently staring down at the crowd—but more strangely—looking straight at *us* baring their teeth in wicked grins.

"Nancy, look at those dogs!" Mark said.

I looked to where he was pointing. "Wow!" They gave me chills.

"They're so ominous-looking," Mark said in a deeper, slower than normal voice. "Take a picture. They look like the dogs of death. The kind you would see at the gates of hell. The watchers!"

I agreed with him as to how evil they looked and snapped a picture. They were silent, but their aggressive stance revealed a dastardly growl that stirred deep inside. They stood at the edge of the building as if they were going to fall off—or pounce. Counter the lovely horse dancing we'd seen just minutes before against the evil dogs. What an eerie contradiction. They made our skin crawl. We kept our eyes on them as we made our way to the restaurant until they were out of sight. Thankfully, they stayed put.

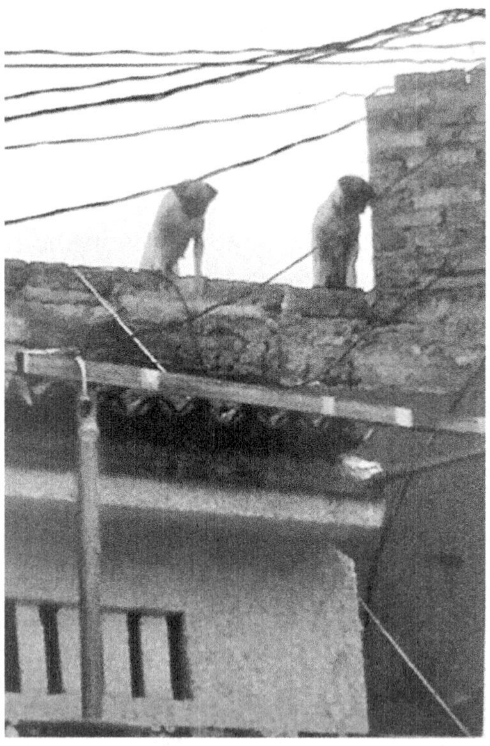

Dogs on rooftop

We made it to the restaurant and Kirk was right, their fish tacos were the best we'd ever had. I needed to use the restroom and made the climb up a narrow spiral staircase to the second floor and found the bathroom made for tiny people with a low, low ceiling—like a small closet. At 5'1½" I had to stoop to be in there. Not only was it tiny—it had to have been one hundred degrees or more in there. Stifling hot. Mark had to go to the bathroom too, and I found it hilarious imagining him struggling in that sauna-hot tiny room with his 6'5" muscular build. Like fitting into the proverbial clown car. His shoulders were so broad he barely made it up the staircase. I don't know how he fit in that bathroom, but he was always good at adapting.

After dinner, we decided to walk to the carnival just down the road before heading back to the bungalow. We ambled around the grounds people-watching and playing typical carnival games and winning little trinkets. Then we happened upon an interesting one for adults. It was a beer bottle breaking game. Stacked next to the game was a giant pile of small rocks. Almost as if someone had a forklift scoop of common everyday rocks and dumped it on the ground. We paid thirty pesos, approximately $1.60, in return for three rocks to throw at empty beer bottles placed upside down on sticks and tried to break them. For every bottle we broke we would get a beer. A person could potentially win three beers for about a dollar and a half. The thing is—it's not so easy to do. Mark had played softball for years and knew how to throw a ball, but his first throw didn't even make it to the bottles. It was so funny. Time and time again he tried to break a bottle, but he never did. We couldn't believe it. We teased him, but he didn't care. He did *not* have a care in the world on that trip.

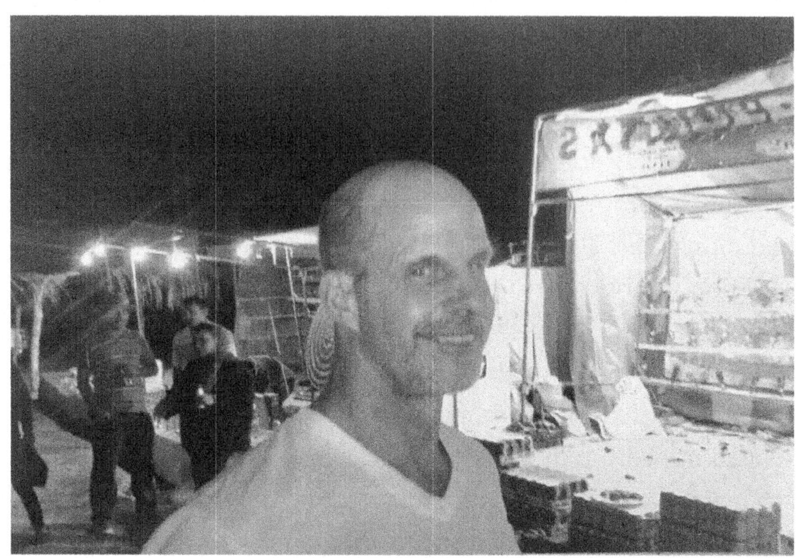

Mark in front of the bottle bash game

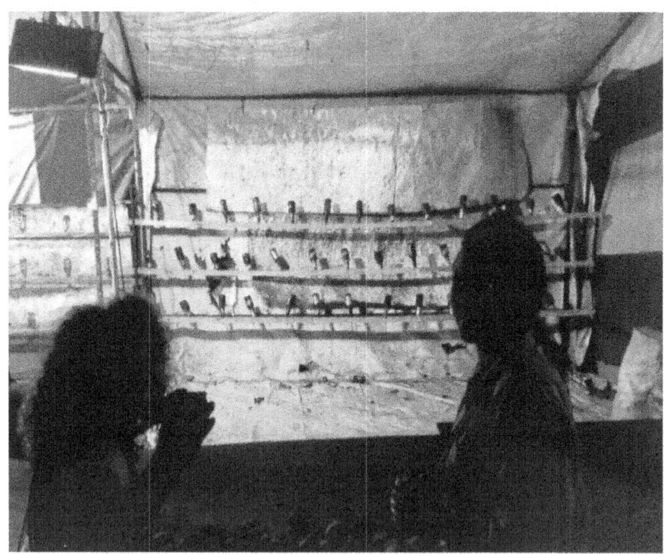

Me (left) and Liz (right) at the bottle bash game.

The four of us ended our second evening in paradise at the bungalow doing the same thing we did the night before. Enjoying each other, our music, and the view and sound of the ocean waves. We went to bed early knowing full well what we were in for on our second day of surfing.

SEVEN

Vacation Day 3—Monday, February 25th

We all woke up ready for the second day of surfing. Sore but ready. Mark commented again about how well he had slept. He told me that two days in a row now, and I thought maybe I'd surprise him with an ocean waves sound machine for our bedroom back home thinking that was the reason why he had slept so well.

The four of us grabbed a banana before heading to the surf school. The same instructors from Sunday were with us in the water on Monday. The instructors and Kirk were right. All the attempts of the previous day to get on the board and stay on it helped in our efforts on Monday. Don't get me wrong. We didn't suddenly breeze past the white-water and pop up on the board. No. There was still plenty of struggle, but we felt more confident. It's incredible the amount of strength it takes to push yourself up and try to pop up to standing position. It was tiring. Every time we fell, we would have to paddle back through the white-water to calmer waters. And for me, it got to the point where I didn't want to catch a wave because once I popped up, I would immediately fall off into the water. It challenged all of us, except for Kirk, but Mark, Liz, and I kept at it.

Just like the day before, we managed to break the basic rules of surfing. Don't grab the rails—you can't balance. Don't bring knees onto the board—you will lose your balance and be thrown off the board. Don't bring your front foot forward first—your feet will land too far back on the board, and you will fall. Don't lock your knees—standing straight compromises the balance, and you will fall. Don't bend your body forward at the waist to balance—you will fall. Don't dive off the board when falling. Jump out as far away from it as possible so it doesn't hit you. Not hit me! The board beat up my body not only from me trying to climb onto it, but by it hitting me nearly every time I fell off. My Sunday bruises started birthing new bruises on Monday.

After numerous tries we finally made it through the white-water and were able to pop up and ride in on a wave. I'm not sure how many times Mark and Liz were able to do it, but I rode in only about three times.

Sadly, after about an hour Mark ended up getting seasick from trying so hard. He had a headache and felt nauseous and dizzy, so we called it quits. Mark always had to make sure he had a full stomach because of his active metabolism, but since he only ate a banana before we surfed that day, we figured his sickness was a result of low blood sugar in combination with all the exertion in the water and on the board. We walked straight to a hut selling drinks on the beach and ordered him a refreshing pineapple drink with lots of ice. Then, we walked to the village and into a restaurant called, Choco Banana, and Mark ordered a chocolate shake, which was unusual, as I'd never seen him order a chocolate shake before, so it appeared that his blood sugar really was low. We all then walked back to the bungalow.

Mark and Kirk wanted to hang at the bungalow and relax, so while they stayed back, Liz and I walked to the village and shopped and had appetizers at a restaurant we happened upon called, Medusa. We were curious to see what a restaurant with that name would look like on the inside thinking it was named after the Greek mythological goddess, Medusa, with living venomous snakes in place of her hair, but it turned out to be named after medusa which is the scientific name for jellyfish. It was an enchanting restaurant off the beaten path fittingly decorated with artwork and hangings of jellyfish in various shapes, sizes, and bright colors.

The two of us had a fun time together, but we missed our guys, so we headed back to the bungalow. On the way back we came across a playful Italian restaurant that had swing chairs hung from poles at the outside bar, and more chairs that hung from trees around the grounds to sit on while being served food and drinks. We found it fascinating and thought it would be fun for the four of us to have dinner there on one of the nights.

When we got back to the bungalow, Mark and Kirk were well rested and ready to walk to an Irish pub on the beach that Kirk knew about. I thought it was ridiculously funny that here we were on the most authentic Mexican trip we'd ever taken, in a small rural village, and one of the beach restaurants was, of all places, an Irish pub. I once again placed my phone and speakers in my purse to listen to our songs as we walked the beach.

We got to the Irish pub and climbed an extremely steep and narrow wooden stairway with no railing up to the rooftop deck. A good-sized crowd was hanging out with many playing cornhole on several boards around the deck. Music played on low volume from the deck speakers with poor sound quality, so I pulled the speakers out of my purse and set them on a table for all to hear. The others on the deck loved it. We played cornhole, sipped beer, and enjoyed the music. It was heavenly. We saw people quickly rush to the edge of the deck and point out to the ocean. We looked out and got to witness a rare opportunity. There were a couple of humpback whales close to the shore repeatedly breaching—jumping out of the water, flipping over, and crashing back down. We stood captivated and were told they only appear in that area from December to March as they look for a place to reproduce before returning to the Arctic. What a wild and wacky thing to experience. Tossing bags in a hole on a warm breezy day, listening to great music and watching whales play from a restaurant rooftop—not a Mexican restaurant, but an Irish pub—on a quaint Mexican beach 2,000 miles away from the cold north winds back home.

The rooftop had no restroom, so Liz and I made our way carefully down the steep stairway with no rails to the main restaurant. While we waited our turn, we watched a surfing show playing on the big screen in the bar. We stood in awe of the talented surfers riding the waves and then realized it was a documentary about world famous surfers who had died while surfing. And I thought, *Wow, I never imagined people dying or drowning while surfing. I thought it was all fun and games.*

After a couple of hours of whale watching, playing cornhole, and watching the sun set at the Irish pub, we headed back to the bungalow and listened to our music and again gazed out at the now full moon lighting up the ocean. We went to bed extra early as Mark and Kirk told us about their plan for the next day. While Liz and I had been in town, Kirk and Mark had arranged with the surf school for the four of us to go to a calmer, easier beach the next day as Mark was determined to get up, and stay up, on a board. We needed to get up early because going to the other beach required a scheduled shuttle bus ride that left right away in the morning. Liz and I looked blankly at each other. We were so tattered and tired from our second day attempts at surfing that we wanted to take a darn day off. That is what we wanted to do, but by gosh, we were not going to say that to Kirk and Mark. So we went to bed that night knowing we'd be heading to another beach the next morning.

EIGHT

Vacation Day 4—Tuesday, February 26th

When we woke up that Tuesday morning, Mark was up and ready for the trip to the easier beach. He again commented about what a wonderful night's sleep he had and how great he felt. That was now the third morning in row he mentioned that. I found it odd that he never raved about a good night's sleep before. Not at home, and not at any of the hotels we'd stayed in over the years. And I thought, *Holy crap, these beds are not that comfortable. In fact, they're kind of hard...and uncomfortable.* It could have been that his knee replacement had helped lessen the strain on his back. It was all part of the *oh my gosh* experience. All of it so wonderful in this extraordinary place and this man of mine was getting his best night's sleep ever. I was so happy for him.

But Kirk, poor Kirk, he had woken up with stomach issues—Montezuma's Revenge was in the house. Even though there were reservations for a shuttle to the other beach, the only thing Kirk could see himself doing all day was eating bananas and consuming copious amounts of rehydrating liquids to make himself feel better.

Of course, we felt terrible for Kirk, but honestly, both Liz and I were relieved that without Kirk we wouldn't be going to surf the other beach, and we looked at each other grinning as if saying, *Yes! Now we can just relax and play for the day.*

But, oh no. Not *my* Mark. He understood Kirk's situation as well as Liz and my desire to relax for the day and he was fine with it. He said, "Kirk, I totally understand. It's alright. You just stay put and get better, and Nancy and Liz, you girls do whatever you want today, but I'm going surfing. I'm not going to give up this opportunity. I need to get up, and stay up, on that board."

Liz and I looked at each other and I thought. *What! That's totally not right.* We were positive, without a doubt in our minds, that Mark would postpone going to the other beach and stay back with us. It didn't occur to us that he'd be willing to go by himself.

Kirk stood leaning against the wall, obviously uncomfortable, and told Mark that he was going with him.

The decision was made. The guys were going surfing, and Liz and I were staying back. Soon afterward, the four of us made our way down the beach to the surf school. Liz and I kissed our men, said good-bye, and strolled back to the bungalow. On our walk back we shared how glad we were to have gotten out of the surfing trip and looked forward to a day of relaxation. I told Liz how excited Mark and I were about his retirement and moving forward with getting a place in Arizona for the winter near her and Kirk, and she and I discussed all the fun we were going to have together.

I shared with her how each morning on the trip that Mark had woken up fresh after having slept all night through. She knew of Mark's struggle with his back and other issues. I told her I simply laid next to him there in the bungalow reveling in his joyfulness thinking, *This is awesome! He's so happy to be here in this paradise. He's pain-free. He's sleeping. Everything is perfect!*

Liz and I sat enjoying each other's company relaxing in the sun and people-watching at a beach restaurant next door to the bungalow. The waves that day had been monstrous, and multiple times while sitting in our beach chairs had commented to each other as to how glad we were for not trying to surf that day. I thought the swelling waters had been caused from the gravitational pull of the full moon, but locals we spoke with said the waves seemed more agitated than just from the full moon. The waves even spun unusually in the safe area of the beach at the sandbar and swimmers struggled against the current in the shallower waters.

We watched people stroll along the beach including vendors selling their wares, and after a while a local woman approached us carrying a display of beautiful blankets. Not the classic brightly colored Mexican serape blankets, but uniquely designed and colored hand-made blankets. I immediately spotted one that had the exact earthy jewel tones in our home, almost as if someone made it specifically for us, and I fell in love with it. I had little interest in souvenirs as we had plenty back home from other vacations, and the only items I had from our trip so far were the two necklaces that Mark helped make for me on our first day, so I bought the blanket.

I absolutely enjoy the sun and water, but with my fair skin, I cannot sunbathe without a coverup. I had packed a pretty floral coverup for our trip, but that day I grabbed one of Mark's white XXL V-neck undershirts that came to mid-thigh, and it looked more like an oversized t-shirt dress on me. The rough waves and wind had torn up the beach pushing sand upward creating tall dunes. I couldn't see the water because of the height of the sand dunes. Liz is taller than me, so she sat higher up in her beach chair and was able to see both the beach and the water. Suddenly, Liz stood up grabbing me, "Nancy, what's that?" She pointed out to the water.

I jumped up and saw something on the edge of the water not moving. We both focused in and realized that it was a person.

"You have to go down there!" Liz commanded.

"What do you mean?"

"You have to go down there!" She pushed me toward the water. "You've gotta see what's happening!"

"What, why me?"

"You know CPR!"

As a personal trainer I do know CPR, so I ran down the beach and as I got closer, I saw a man face down in the water and thought, *Oh no, what am I going to find?* I had no idea how long he had been there. No one else was running to this man, but then not many people were around due to the turbulent waves, and maybe other people's views had been blocked like mine had been.

I reached him and saw that he had a board strapped to his ankle and I carefully turned him over on his back. He was unconscious and blood streamed down his battered face. I shook him a little, but no response. He was breathing so I pulled him a little further out of the water and propped him up on my lap. I took off Mark's t-shirt to wipe his face to assess the situation. He must have fallen, and it looked like the board hit him between the eyes on the bridge of his nose because his nose was split wide open oozing clots of blood.

After a minute or so he came to and looked up at me blinking. When he realized his condition he pleaded, "Don't call the police or ambulance! I don't have insurance. They say it's free but it's not. I can't afford it. You're my angel. I'm going to be okay. Just don't call anyone. Please." He spoke English sounding like he was from the USA or Canada.

At that same time Liz had been yelling to the restaurant staff from the beach, "Man down! We need help!"

No one from the restaurant came to help so Liz ran next door inside the bungalow and filled two glasses of fresh water and rushed them down to us. One for the man to drink from and the other for me to clean his bloodied face. We sat there with him for the longest time with no one coming to help. We thought it extremely strange that no one else came to see what was happening.

Finally, after about twenty minutes a man walked over to us. He said, "I'm a doctor. I saw you roll him over and lay him on his back and prop him up. Not many people will step in because of legalities in possibly causing physical harm to an injured person when trying to help them, but I watched nearby and saw that you did everything right."

The doctor had heard the man telling me he didn't have insurance, and that's when he walked down to us at the water's edge. He examined the surfer closely assessing his condition and when he determined the man was okay to walk, he volunteered to take him back to his own bungalow to stitch him up. We all helped the man to his feet and the doctor held onto him as the man limped across the sand. Out of nowhere, a woman appeared saying she knew the man and asked, "What happened to him?"

It was so strange. *Where did she come from, and where was she when he laid face down in the water?*

The man looked to be about seventy years old and she in her early sixties. She told us they met earlier in the day in Nuevo Vallarta and on a whim decided to drive north to Sayulita so he could surf. It was clear they didn't know each other well as she only knew his first name, of which I do not recall.

Liz and I then returned to our beach chairs for a few more hours trying to relax after helping the battered man. At around 4 pm, we spotted Mark and Kirk walking up the beach toward us. I had never seen Mark stride with such animation—his head held high with chest thrown out strutting like a king. His face radiated and I knew that meant he got up on the board. Liz and I were so excited for him, and we stood and cheered for him as the two of them made their way to us.

Mark sat on the edge of my beach chair and noticed the blanket right away, "Hey, that totally matches everything in our house! It's beautiful."

The fact that he commented on it at all was one thing, but for him to notice how well it matched our home décor was another, and that made the blanket even more special.

After a while, the four of us went inside the bungalow and enjoyed some appetizers and the beautiful oceanfront scenery from Kirk and Liz's rooftop. Mark expounded more about his success at the other beach and was still so excited that he had gotten up on the board. He sat proudly like a peacock and his face gleamed.

Kirk then shared a story about a dog that approached them, specifically Mark, earlier that day as they waited for the surf school shuttle. A stray dog, of which there are lots of them in the area, approached Mark and brushed up against his leg. Mark loves dogs so he petted him. A local bystander told them that the dog had a reputation of not really liking or warming up to people, and workers at the school, who knew of the dog, also commented about how unusual it was that the dog had warmed up to Mark and stayed next to him for so long allowing him to pet him. Kirk told us Mark replied to everyone, "Well, you do know what dog spelled backwards is, right?" He grinned playfully and said, "It's G-O-D of course." Kirk said everyone at the school laughed. We all did too.

Mark and Kirk sat facing the sun and Liz and I sat across from them with our backs to the ocean. Out of nowhere Liz bursts out, "Oh my god Mark your eyes are so blue! And your teeth, I didn't know you had such white teeth! It's like you're glowing!"

I looked at him and she was right. He did have beautiful white teeth and deep blue eyes, but at that moment, because he was so delighted that he got up on the board that day, his skin, teeth, and eyes radiated extraordinarily bright.

What a wonderful time. We were all happy sharing lots of laughter in our little slice of paradise and listening to our favorite music playing in the background.

One of the songs on the playlist started and Mark began tapping his feet. He loved the song, but I knew he didn't know the artist. He enjoyed all sorts of music but didn't necessarily know the artists. The song playing was "Need You Now" by Lady Antebellum. We liked to stump him because he was so overly filled with facts of all kinds, so I started joking with him, "Okay Mark, who sings this one?"

He sat taller in his chair and said very matter-of-factly in his resonant voice, "Lady Antebellum."

"No way! How could you possibly know that?" I teased back. And we all laughed some more.

We continued razzing and joking with one another. It was close to 5 pm when Mark and Kirk said they wanted to get in a final session of body surfing, not board surfing, before the four of us got showered and changed to walk to the fun Italian swing chair restaurant that Liz and I had stumbled upon the day before. Liz and I said sure, and that we wanted to go and watch them, but that neither of us felt like body surfing.

The waves in front of the bungalow were too choppy and dangerous for body surfing, so we walked about a hundred yards north where we could see that the waves were perfect for it. The north beach normally has far fewer people because it is further away from the busier southside of the beach which is closer to the village where we'd taken our surfing lessons. By that time of day, we had the beach to ourselves as it was dinner time for most people so no one else was around us. When our guys headed for the water, Liz and I settled down on a hilly spot on the sand as the best place to watch them. I brought along the new blanket I'd purchased earlier in the day for Liz and me to sit on, but it was a bit windy and cool, so she and I wrapped ourselves in it instead.

Liz and I chatted as we watched Mark and Kirk walk into the water together and stand in waist-high water waiting for the first wave to come in. The waves mushroomed and rolled making them perfect for body surfing.

The guys were about an arm's length away from each other when they caught the first wave and body surfed back into shore. They were having a ball whooping it up in the surf. Liz and I just watched and laughed. The guys walked back out together and stood again at about an arm's length from each other, but this time in only about thigh-high water waiting for another perfect wave. Then, in an instant, Mark ended up about fifty feet away from Kirk and further out in the water.

Liz and I looked at each other puzzled wondering how Mark got from point A to point B so rapidly—in a split second. Mark was now in at least neck high water or maybe even treading, and he had a distressed look on his face as if thinking, *Uh, oh, I shouldn't be out here.*

Liz and I quickly stood up. Both of us were confused by what had just happened and I yelled and waved to Kirk to get his attention and pointed out to Mark.

Kirk looked to where I was pointing much further away from where he himself stood in thigh-high water and motioned Mark toward shore yelling, "Old Sac, get your ass back in here!"

Mark heard him, waved, and yelled back, "Okay!"

Liz and I saw the next set of waves coming. They frightened us. They were suddenly bigger and more intense than the previous sets. Scary big. It did not look good at all. My heart raced and I thought, *He's going to get hurt.*

The waves swelled and rapidly billowed higher and higher behind Mark. He didn't see what was behind him. Kirk was far enough away from Mark that he wasn't going to get hit in the same way that Mark was about to. It all happened so fast. Then crash! The giant crest of a wave came straight down on Mark. Then right away another wave and then another. There was no settling between the crests.

Liz and I darted toward the water. I pictured Mark in the merciless waves being tossed around like a ragdoll pummeled by the upheaval into the sand. I thought when he surfaced, he'd come out totally annoyed and cursing the ocean with sand in his mouth, ears, eyes, and who knows where else.

I waited for him to surface. A few seconds passed. The sunlight pierced upon the chaotic waves making it impossible to see anything. More seconds passed. No sign of Mark. Then many more seconds without seeing him.

Kirk yelled, "Don't take your eyes off him!"

I yelled back, "We don't see him!"

Liz and I sprinted up and back, crisscrossing each other trying to see any sign of Mark. Kirk desperately searched for a surfboard or a buoy, but there were none nearby as we were not around other people, and the surf school was about a half-mile down the beach. There was no time to run and get a board. We needed to stay focused on where Mark went under.

We cupped our hands above our eyes to try to see out into the harshly sunlit billowing and crashing waves, but we could not see him. Mark wasn't out that far when he went under, but the waves had become so tumultuous that it would have been suicide for any one of us to swim out and attempt to rescue him without a safety device like a board or a buoy.

Noooooo! This can't be happening! No way! No way in hell!

Liz and I ran up and down the beach, while Kirk stayed in the area yelling and hoping residents nearby would hear him to try to get a board in the water.

Kirk kept yelling, "Don't take your eyes off him!"

Liz and I shouted back, "We don't see him! We never saw him surface!"

Liz ran up and back toward the water vehemently screaming, "No way! No way!" Desperately shouting, "No way!" Feverishly screaming and cursing, "No way! No way!"

Pandemonium permeated the air. There were no decent words to describe the turmoil and confusion in those hellish seconds upon seconds and relentlessly agonizing minutes. All I could think as we frantically navigated the beach was, *This is not real! This cannot be real! This is not happening!*

Liz and I decided to split up along the beach, while Kirk ran about a half-mile past the surf school to the south end to see how to get a boat in the water. The local fishermen were done fishing for the day. Their boats sat high up on the beach away from the tide which required a vehicle to tow them into the water, and there were no recreational watercraft like jet-skis around. It was a small, remote, mellow fishing and surf village. There were no commercial or private docks with boats tied to them either—it was the open ocean. Besides a small fishing boat, the most you could get in the water was a surfboard, but it was too dangerous as the ebb and flow never settled. It was thunderous. The only way to get a boat in the water was to hire a fisherman, so Kirk ran several more yards to the village to find a bilingual fisherman or a bilingual local to translate. It was so anguishly paralyzing seeing the boats readily available but with no one there to get one in the water.

Suddenly, out of nowhere, I saw two surfers clutching their boards rushing toward me. They must have heard the screaming and yelling. They reached me and one of them pointed to the southside of the beach hollering above the noisy wind and waves, "We're going to go in, we're going to try to cut him off!" I was relieved that he spoke English.

I argued back, motioning to the north, "No, he went in over there! He's not going to go that way. He's going to go toward the rocks!"

"No, no, lady you have to understand, the current flows south! And the waters are calmer there so it's safe for us to get a board in."

"But he was swept off to the north!" I insisted.

I saw where the wave struck Mark and figured he was treading water with the current sweeping him toward the rocks—huge boulders the size of cars. My fear was that the turbulent waves would overtake him pushing him into the crashing surf and onto the boulders. I ran to the north to see if he was heading for the boulders while Liz ran south where the surfers planned to search. I thought, *Ok, fine. They know their stuff about the current, but I know what I saw.*

I ran a good distance and made it about halfway to the boulders and stopped. I stood on the beach for several minutes searching against the blinding sunlit water yelling out for Mark. Then, I looked back to the south and saw one of the boarders in the water raising and waving his arm, so I tore across the sand over there. My mind racing, *Oh my god, they see him, they found him, they have him! He must have been treading water all this time. Oh my god! Thank you.* I was so relieved and so grateful. I stood next to Liz. I struggled to catch my breath; my arms wrapped tightly against my chest.

We watched as the boarders paddled in, but I didn't see Mark and thought maybe he was hanging onto the back of one of the boards.

A crowd had gathered, and I asked, "They have him, right?"

A woman standing next to us said no, the hand signal meant he and the other boarder did *not* see him.

I dropped to my knees. I thought, *No way, this can't be happening!*

Shortly afterward, a snowbird approached us saying, "I'm sorry. Many of us have had eyes on the water since we first heard the yelling, and we haven't seen him at all. The waves were so constant and big against the blinding sunlight that we just couldn't see well enough at the water."

Near-drownings occur frequently there, and when locals hear upheaval on the beach, they are set and ready to grab their binoculars and 'get eyes on the water' to help search for people in trouble.

Suddenly, something arose within me. I had to keep my wits about me. I had to move beyond the panic mode that consumed me. While Kirk attempted to get a fishing boat in the water, Liz and I decided to continue searching down the southside of the beach. We rushed further down the beach about a half-mile to the sandbar. It is the farthest part of the beach to safely walk before reaching the surf that swirled against other large boulders jutting out into the ocean making it dangerous to access. But Liz and I thought maybe Mark made it ashore and was possibly injured and stranded in the rocky area, so we eased our way bare foot around the slippery and sharp rocks in ankle to knee-deep water confident that we would find him there. We stumbled up, over, and around the hazardous terrain calling out Mark's name for a long while but we didn't see or hear him. We heard a loud noise on the beach and looked over to see a truck towing a fishing boat into the water several yards away from us, so we worked our way back out of the rocks and ran to watch the truck release the boat into the ocean.

It was about 6:30 pm by that time—over an hour since Mark had disappeared. Kirk, Liz, and I watched anxiously as the boat captain and two helpers zigzagged in the water searching for Mark. They stayed out for about thirty minutes before arriving back on the beach. As Kirk, Liz, and I approached the boat, the captain shook his head. He was a resident Spanish speaker, and with the help of a snowbird who translated for us, the captain said they didn't see any sign of Mark, and since it was nearing sunset, they needed to call off the search. He confirmed what the surfers had told us, saying the currents in that area move southward so the search would continue in that area the next morning.

A local police officer who spoke limited English approached us, and with the same snowbird translating, confirmed what the captain said explaining that it was too dark to continue a search and promised it would resume first thing in the morning saying, "No se preocupe, habrá personas aquí para ayudarla." (Don't worry there will be people here to help you.) "Estaremos peinando la playa." (We will be combing the beach.) "Tendremos botes en el agua." (We will have boats in the water.)

And it took me a few seconds for me to realize what they were saying, and I thought, *Okay. I get it. But wait a minute! No, no, no!*

I waved my hands at the water and shouted at the officer in a hell no tone of voice, "Are you kidding me! You're saying you're going to leave my husband out there in the ocean? You know he's out there! Now you're telling me it's 7:15 at night and there won't be people searching until sunrise tomorrow morning, when he is out there fighting for his life right now? Injured maybe! Lying on the beach somewhere! We know he's still alive, but is he going to be able to survive the night out there in the waves? On the beach? In the cold? I don't understand—don't you have boats with search lights to be out looking for him, or searchers with flashlights looking for him on the shore?"

The translator told the police officer what I said, and the officer lowered his eyes to the sand and responded, "Lo siento mucho Señora."

(I'm very sorry ma'am.) "Esta muy oscuro afuera." (It is too dark outside.) Mañana. (Tomorrow.) "Lo prometo." (I promise.)

I looked at them horrified. My mind whirled trying to take in everything so opposite of what I was expecting to hear. I fell again to my knees and put my head in my hands, my whole body shook. I know the officer probably didn't know exactly what I'd said, and I could tell that the translator only gave him the gist of it, but he certainly understood the fury and frustration in my voice and the urgency of the situation. *Didn't he? Didn't they?*

The officer spoke with such nonchalance as if to say, "Okay little lady calm down now, all will be fine. You just go back to your bungalow, get some rest and all will be better in the morning when we return to help."

Kirk, Liz, and I slogged back to the bungalow in a mired state of shock and uncertainty forced to wait until morning. I could hear voices around us, but everything was distorted. Words reverberated as if my brain were caught inside a metal can with the words of others heard but not comprehended because all my brain could handle was the immediacy of the situation—my mind buzzed and swirled.

As the three of us despondently inched along the sand, the same woman who had told us the meaning of the boarder's hand signal approached us saying she was sorry, and handed me my blanket that I had left on the northside of the beach.

It was around 9 pm when I suddenly realized, *Oh my god, I have to call our children. What the hell! I have to call and tell them their dad is missing and I have no idea where he is.* What an unconscionable thing to think about. I vacillated in a muddled state of disbelief that Mark was even missing and wondered if I really needed to call them at all. I truly thought he was alive. True, he was not there with us, and that reality was mind boggling, but I did *not* believe he was dead. But I had to make the phone call. But what was I supposed to say? In my spirit, I believed Mark was going to come walking up at any moment wounded and fuming mad that we were just sitting around while he made his way back in the dark— barefoot, cold, and *hungry* demanding, "Where were you!"

My hands were sweating and shaking as I picked up my cell phone. It was warm where I was, around 75 degrees on the Pacific Coast, but I felt chilled to the bone as if I were back home in the frigid 25-degree weather. Oddly enough the time zone is the same in both Minnesota and Sayulita.

I called our son Jacob, but he didn't answer his phone. He had been staying back and forth between his house and ours while we were gone. I was so distraught and didn't want to wait around for Jacob, so I called our son, Lucas.

"Lucas, this is mom, where is your brother?" I could hear my voice shaking and weak, like I had swallowed it.

"He's not here."

I tried to remain cool and calm and spoke slower than normal. "Lucas I need to talk to Jacob. He's not answering. I need to get a hold of him."

"I think he's at his house."

"Lucas, he's not answering his phone. I need you to go over to his house and get him on the phone. I need to talk to Jacob. I have some news about your dad."

"What do you mean about dad?"

"Lucas I need to talk to Jacob."

"What do you mean? Why can't you tell *me*?"

He was bucking me and fighting me back and forth and wouldn't help me out and go get Jacob. He couldn't understand why it was so necessary to get Jacob, so he was battling me.

Eventually, I couldn't do it anymore and I started crying. I desperately demanded, "I need you to get your brother to the house because something has happened. I need for you, Jacob, and Sami to be together." That's what I think I said, something like that, that something has happened. And he just kept fighting me. And finally, I said, "Lucas, your dad is missing."

"*Who* is this? Who *are* you? I don't believe you! Why would you say something like that?"

"Lucas this is your mother."

"No, it's not! This isn't my mom. Who is this?"

And that's all I remember of the conversation. After the phone call home, Kirk, Liz, and I sat outside in the dimly lit area of the bungalow for hours upon hours anguishly waiting. Waiting for my Mark. Waiting for the sun to rise in ten hours. We sat. We meandered. Looking out toward the ocean was like peering into an otherworldly abyss. With the exception of the waning full moon shining on the water, there was only pitch darkness out there. Soul-stealing eeriness consumed me as I looked out into the blackness toward the water believing Mark was treading water or beached somewhere injured. I sat curled up on a chair in the outside corner of the covered patio wrapped in the big blanket I bought earlier that day on the beach, which now seemed so very, very long ago. I didn't want to lay down in the bed because I believed Mark was alive and going to walk up any moment mad as hell, or maybe he was out in the water hanging on to something desperately trying to make his way to shore. I thought if Mark was not sleeping, I was not going to sleep either. It would have been impossible for me to do so anyway. My punctured heart throbbed—a vile foreign feeling I had never experienced in my life. A constant stabbing. A ruthless blistering like chemical acid churning and burning in my chest. My stomach gritty, feeling like I swallowed a glass of sand. My mind was caught in a malicious replay of the moment that Mark disappeared. At one point, I wandered into the bedroom and sat in agony on the floor leaning against the bed trying to escape the loud waves. I called my friend Kim back home, uncontrollably crying and muttering that we couldn't find Mark, and that we had to wait until morning for the search to continue.

Liz and Kirk remained with me on the main level in the tiny space of the bungalow. We went over and over the mayhem with each other bewildered as to how this could have happened. Mark was less than fifty feet from shore when he went under. There was nothing anyone could do. It was impossible—we *could not* help him. We *could not* fix it. There was nothing, absolutely nothing we could do. There we were…in a foreign land with officials who spoke little to no English, and no emergency aid like there would have been back home. That level of helplessness is something I had never felt before nor could have ever imagined. The three of us—hazy-minded and caught up in confusion—could only shake our heads in disbelief. We looked at each other; beyond each other, all captured in the hell of the imprisonment of powerlessness. We blurted out anguished frustrations over and over, and continually uttered, "This is unbelievable!" Besides those few words, there was little conversation. We just waited. Paced. Ruminated. Haphazardly prayed—begging God for Mark's return. I wanted to transcend my body into a giant osprey, a native bird in the area, whose night vision would allow me to see into the blackness and fly to find Mark and pull him from the sea or retrieve him from a nearby shore. I did not belong there simply waiting. Mark did not belong wherever he was either. What a cruel, dehumanizing struggle to have to endure. In the United States there would have been helicopters, boats, and divers with searchlights tirelessly scouring the area for a lost swimmer in the dark.

After a few hours, I told Kirk and Liz it was okay for them to go upstairs to their loft as I just wanted to be alone in my thoughts while waiting for Mark, but they were so kind and stayed with me until around 3 am. At that time, I thought I would try laying down in the bed and Liz asked if I wanted her to sleep with me. I thanked her but said no. She and Kirk then climbed to their loft. I laid wide-eyed in bed for a very short time before I got back up. I moved from wandering in circles around the bungalow to sitting and rocking on the bed, and back to curling myself in a ball in the outside chair impatiently waiting for the sunrise and rescue workers to arrive.

Mark had taken off his regular shorts and shoes and wore only his swim trunks when he went into the water. His shorts were laying on the bed where he left them, and I picked them up, brought them on the chair with me and hugged them tightly to my chest like they were a pillow. His shoes stayed exactly where he left them by the door with his socks sticking out of each one as he had always done before. Whenever we played beach volleyball or hung on a beach somewhere on vacation, Mark regularly put his wallet in one shoe and car keys in the other shoving both toward the toe of each shoe. He would then stuff his socks into each one thinking no one was going to want to touch stinky socks and would leave the shoes alone. I could not touch or move them because I thought if I did it would be to Mark's demise, like a bad omen, so I left them alone because I believed he was coming back for them.

I could not block out the sound of the waves. What otherwise would have been a sweetly soothing sound became an uncompromising bellowing as each set of waves crashed on the sand just a few yards away. And I could only think, *Mark, where are you?*

Mark was a strong swimmer. I'm not sure how much swimming he did as a child, but I do know that when he started working at Xcel Energy at age nineteen, he played on the company softball team, and they made it to nationals every year primarily traveling to the Florida coast for the playoffs. When not playing ball, the team headed to the ocean to swim, boogie board, and body surf. Mark was always about fitness and preparation. To ready himself for swimming for our vacations or the baseball playoffs he'd see how long he could hold his breath while driving. Or when watching a television show or movie, he'd mimic someone underwater having to hold their breath to survive. And it wasn't just in preparation for swimming. Mark routinely practiced holding his breath as part of his workouts to keep his lungs strong. He always challenged himself to go beyond the norm. He didn't like to dismiss something as normal or average. If someone said something about the average this or that, he'd ask what that had to do with him. "What's your point?" he'd say. And he encouraged others asking what 'average' had to do with them as well urging, "Why strive for normal?" His body and lungs were so strong that when body surfing, he could plank his body so well that he was able to ride the waves longer than others, and people admired his ability.

As I continued sitting balled up in the chair outside, I could close my eyes but not my ears. Not that I slept at all, but I could not smother the sound of the waves by shutting windows as there were none to shut in our open-air bungalow. No insulated glass, no soundproof headphones to silence the sound of waves hitting the shore. Pillows around my ears offered no help either. The few seconds between the recurrent ebb of the waves outward and the crescendo of the flow inward nearly drove me mad.

The slow, swooshing sounds that the four of us had yearned for and experienced the previous three nights as a reprieve from the cold winter back home no longer brought comfort. The other nights we listened to peaceful waves lapping as if saying, "Relax, relax, relax." It's the reason why multitudes of people around the world flock to the beaches of the world. It's why lovers stroll slowly along the beach at night together. It's to allow the sound of non-threatening ocean waves ease us into a place of contentment. Now they sounded like unusually threatening waves mercilessly hissing, roaring, and crashing. Void of all tranquility. A deafening incessant disturbance of swelling, shrinking, and sighing. Whooshing, smashing, and churning. With an overriding hollow haunting whisper taunting me over, and over, and over again.

At times, the waves sounded more like unceasing distant rumbling thunder. Other times like the sound of a nearby roadway with the unyielding sound of approaching and fading traffic rushing, rumbling, and hushing—overpowering every other sound around. But the thunder never moved on and the traffic never stopped. And it wasn't just the sound. I could smell its brininess and feel its vibration. When the waves crashed, they sent unremitting shock waves rippling through my body at the bungalow only a few yards away. And I thought *Mark, I know you made it. Make your way to us. The bungalow lights are on. We are awake waiting for you.*

Time was my enemy that night as I continued sitting scrunched up in the dark listening to the antagonistic waves. My chest felt weighted like a lead vest had been place upon it suppressing every agonizing breathe in and breathe out. I just wanted *my* Mark to walk up. Uninjured or injured, angry or not angry, it didn't matter, I just wanted him back at the bungalow.

My phone pinged. It was our daughter Sami sending me a text. Simple texts with few words. *Hi mom, are you awake? I love you. What are you doing? How are you feeling? What are you thinking?*

The gripping emotional pain made me physically ill. Dealing with Mark's disappearance while being separated from my children after telling them their dad was missing devastated me. But I needed to keep my wits about me for myself so I could be strong for them while striving with all my might to solely concentrate on finding Mark.

That mission was at the forefront of my thinking as my mind continually replayed the terrible moment the first and two subsequent waves crashed down on him searing the otherwise unimaginable visual into my soul. But it was not unimaginable. I saw it happen. The voracious waves were like a tyrannical enemy, heartlessly calloused toward Mark's indefensible position—falsely arresting him, tearing him from our grasp— now a prisoner of the sea. For every barbarous wave that forced its way upon the shore I wondered, *Was that the wave that brought him ashore?*

NINE

Remembering When We Met

With my mind wandering and reeling in a mangled mess, thoughts surfaced back to when Mark and I first met. It was 1984, and I was nineteen years old and had just moved to Minneapolis from Grand Forks, North Dakota. I worked as an allocation clerk for Investors Diversified Services (IDS). The IDS Center is still the tallest building in downtown Minneapolis with fifty-seven stories, and I worked on the 26th floor where I enjoyed spectacular views of the city and surrounding parks and lakes. In comparison, the town of Grand Forks had one escalator. That was about as equivalent as a person moving from Minneapolis to New York City where some of the buildings nearly double the height of the IDS Center. It was a big deal. I was lucky enough to live with my sister, Kathy, and her husband, Woody, and their two daughters for six months until I got an apartment of my own.

Mark and Woody both worked at Xcel Energy—Mark as a lineman and Woody in customer service. Both of them played on the work softball team, and Kathy and Woody invited me along to one of their games, so I put on my snakeskin cowboy boots, jeans, and a t-shirt and went to the game. There was room in the bleachers with older people, but at age nineteen, happy-go-lucky, and working in the big city; I wanted to see and be seen apart from the others, so I perched myself on top of a green metal storage container behind the backstop and had a terrific view of the field. I noticed Mark in the outfield and remembered meeting him briefly the previous year at one of their games when I had visited Kathy and Woody.

My desire to sit separately in order to stand out from the crowd worked in my favor. During their inning at bat, Mark walked over to me, and we exchanged small talk. I went to the next three games and then afterward with everyone to a local bar that sponsored the team. Mark and I talked a bit at the bar, and we hit it off nicely.

After the third game, Mark was so charming, he asked Woody if it was okay if he asked me to drive to the bar with him, as he was thirty, and mindful of our eleven-year age difference and what others might think. Woody knew of Mark's solid reputation and said yes.

I thought it was very polite of Mark to ask Woody, so I said yes and drove to the bar with him. Mark and I got to know one another better that night and it was then that he asked me out on a date. On our first date, we went to the original historical Broadway Pizza in Minneapolis along the scenic Mississippi River. Mark ordered his favorite large pizza with their renowned cracker-style crust, and then sweetly looked at me and in his unwavering baritone voice asked, "And…. what would you like?"

He caught me off guard, and I thought, *Are you kidding me? He's going to eat a large pizza by himself?* But I could tell he was serious, so I quickly looked at the menu and ordered a hoagie. I ate most of mine and had leftovers to bring home, but he ate his entire pizza at the restaurant. There were never any leftovers for him to take home. And back then, a large pizza was more like an extra-large pizza by today's standards.

We continued dating, and the first time I cooked for Mark, I told him what I was planning to make which included a side dish of corn. He asked me if I would call his mom and ask for her special corn recipe. I thought it was a strange request, *a special corn recipe?* I'd met his mother, but we'd only been around each other a couple of times. Mark gave me her phone number, so I called and told her I was cooking for Mark and that he asked me to call for her corn recipe. There was silence on the other end for a few seconds—then a big belly laugh. She could hardly speak she was laughing so hard. "So, you would like the special recipe?"

I was embarrassed. I thought Mark had set me up for something. "Yes, Mark told me you make the best corn."

It turns out in the earlier days, when his mom made large family dinners for the holidays, the last item she placed in the oven was a corn casserole topped with lots of butter, salt, and pepper where she inevitably forgot about it. When she finally realized it was in the oven, the butter had created a nice brown burnt crust on top. Mark loved it like that and for all his years growing up he thought it was her intentional *special* recipe.

Early into our dating we discovered that we both had a great sense of adventure and challenged one another's creativity and intellect. We discovered we were like-minded spiritually, that we each cared about the well-being of others, and realized the importance of the family bond. We treasured our own meaningful friendships outside of our relationship, and over time valued the melding of those friendships with our family at various social gatherings.

Our eleven-year age difference was never an issue for us. Although some people were curious about it since Mark was more seasoned and settled than me, and I was in the final year of my teens and living a bit more carefree. But we hit it off. We reveled in our similarities and inspired each other through our differences. Mark had always described me as an old soul and that it seemed like I was closer to *his* age. I was never a giggly type of girl. I considered myself as a strong independent person, and I never felt that I *needed* someone. I did have a long, loving relationship before I met Mark, and it was good, but it ended when I moved to Minneapolis.

After living on my own in my own apartment, I woke up one night with an *aha* moment knowing no one else was responsible for what I had right then and there. I never put myself in a position to ever ask my dad, mom, or anyone else for help. And that for me was a valuable thing to realize—that I'd become self-sufficient. I didn't own a car at that time and took the bus to work and elsewhere. I paid my bills and had enough to spare, and I believe that was the combination that drew Mark and I together—both of us hardworking, financially independent people with a passion for adventure.

By nature, Mark liked and needed his space and freedom and was the type of person that took a while to commit, but once he was in, he was in all the way. I'm similar in that way of being in all the way once I commit, but in contrast, am more of an outgoing, impulsive dreamer ready for the next journey either on my own or taking others along for the ride. I delight in the mysteries of life whereas Mark, though adventurous, liked things more defined. He hated it when I presented a 'what if' fanciful type of hypothetical scenario, and he'd question, "Well that isn't the way it is. So why would you be presenting that idea?"

Our strong points that allowed us to work well together were our own gifts of communication and imagination, mine idealistic, his realistic; our positive outlook on life and interest toward the immaterial things in life—the important intangible things. We shared a strong Christian faith, and our equally strong wills made for interesting conversations and debates. When we disagreed or argued about the things that couples struggle through, we did so with respect avoiding any mudslinging or regrets.

A year-and-a-half into dating, Mark and I were driving to Broadway Pizza where we had gone to on our first date, and where we'd been many times since, and he pulled over before we got there. It was in an industrial area, and I thought he wanted to park and make out, but he had a serious look on his face, and at first didn't say anything. I got nervous since he didn't reach over to kiss me. Then very soberly, and even a bit anxiously, he asked me to marry him. I really thought it was going to be a different kind of something serious. He told me he'd been so confident about us and that he knew he was going to marry me the moment he met me. I felt the same and said, "Yes!"

We made it to our favorite restaurant to celebrate another significant time in our relationship, and one of the first things Mark said is that we needed to find a house to start our lives together because his duplex was located in a tougher part of the city.

Together Mark and I told his parents about the engagement, and he asked me not to tell anyone else until after we told my parents. Mark and my dad shared a special bond as they both worked for the same energy company, but in two separate cities, and different capacities. A couple of days later, Mark flew both of us to Grand Forks for the day to visit my parents, which is a four-and-a-half-hour drive from Minneapolis, but only an hour-and-twenty-minute flight. He took my dad aside in a back room in their home and asked him for my hand in marriage, and my dad said yes.

About a month later, we met with a jeweler friend of Mark's to design an engagement ring. I told Mark I only needed a gold band, but he insisted on a diamond.

We had a seven-month engagement, and in that time we found a house and closed in August. The house seemed too big for the two of us, so we invited Mark's sister, Missy, to live in the basement apartment, but I didn't move in until two months later after our wedding on Friday, October 17, 1986, nearly two years after we started dating.

Our wedding was held on a mild 60-degree day. I was honored to have worn my mother's wedding dress, and Mark had flown me home a couple of times beforehand for the fittings. We were married in the year of my dad and mom's 30th wedding anniversary. Mark had agreed to get married in my hometown of Grand Forks in the same big church where my mom and dad had been married. It meant everything to me and my mom that I wore her dress. Our wedding was large and beautiful with over three hundred people. And the photos of our wedding, as compared to my parents' wedding photos with me in mom's dress and standing on the same altar, are stunningly similar. Not only similar. Priceless.

The reception was held in the church basement with a meal and cake. My dad sang and played the drums in a polka band, and he and his bandmates played at the reception and lit up the dance floor.

We planned another reception the next day in Minneapolis as only Mark's parents and a few of his family and friends attended our wedding in Grand Forks. So the next morning people drove down to Minneapolis for the other reception including relatives and longtime friends of Mark's, new friends of mine, and our friends together. The second reception included cake, coffee, an open bar, and a dance.

Both of us were elated to start a new life together as a married couple. I was fortunate to have found someone so special and I give most of the credit to God. Somebody watched over me and gave me guidance that Mark was the right person for me. And he turned out to be a loving man of honesty and integrity.

TEN

Day 5—First Full Day After Mark's Disappearance,
Wednesday, February 27th

At sunrise about 7:30 am, Mark had not returned to the bungalow. Kirk, Liz, and I looked out onto the beach and did not see any officials organizing a search. No police. No boats. Only some local snowbirds we heard talking. I asked Kirk to please go and find out what was happening. He walked out to the group, and I watched all of them as I tried to read their body language.

After several minutes Kirk walked back with his head down.

I thought, *Something is wrong.*

"There's nothing going on," Kirk said.

I snapped. "What do you mean there's nothing going on? We were told. We were *promised!*"

"Well…," he said in a pained whisper, "there's nobody out there except some local snowbirds."

When he told me that, I stormed out onto the beach and raced to the group of people who were mingling and talking about Mark's disappearance.

I demanded, "Where are the searchers? Where are the boats?" I wasn't crying. I was *furious*. In a nutshell, the group told me straight out that there would be no help from the local government in the search.

"What!" I shouted. "You've got to be kidding me!" My arm shot straight out to the ocean. Mark is out there and he's alive in the water or on a beach somewhere! And there's *nothing?*"

Kirk stood beside me, and we wrangled back and forth with the group asking a multitude of questions about what we needed to do and who we needed to go to for help while trying to process their absurd answers about how there would be no help from local officials.

We were beside ourselves. Bewildered. Totally perplexed. *This is insane! This is ridiculous! You've got to be kidding!*

I fired back saying, "I know people in the United States and what channels to go through to get things done, and I know the local media back home, and, and…"

One of the women stopped me and said, "Lady, if you really do know people in the United States and you really do have an in with the media, then you better start making phone calls right now, because they have *no* resources here, they have *no* plan, and *no* intention of doing anything to find your husband. They're simply waiting for him to wash ashore…somewhere."

Done. Conversation over. My brain felt like a gong hit forcefully with a mallet.

She and the rest of the group continued saying, "We're sorry, there are no resources here. Nobody's going to help you."

The owner of the bungalow was part of the group and all he kept saying was, "Oh, he probably had a heart attack."

"Well, no," I fired back, "he didn't have a heart attack, *okay*?"

I then ran back to the bungalow, my thoughts in a whirl. *What's happening? What is this nightmare! No way! Why can't anyone help us?* I grabbed my cell phone and called my friend Kim to have her get the phone number for the US Embassy or Consulate in Mexico, and to please get in touch with her niece, who was my producer at KSTP-TV with the "Twin Cities Live" show back home. I called Kim because I had no idea where to start with getting the help we needed. She reminded me that we had spoken the night before, but I told her I did not remember that call to her.

In our hammering back forth with the locals on the beach, we were reminded that drownings were not an uncommon thing there, but what we did not know is that the local government had no resources to find the missing.

Because of our remote location it forced us to take matters into our own hands. By then I was angry as hell. Real angry. Kim called me back with phone numbers for the US Embassy in Mexico City. For hours on end that morning I was on the phone leaving messages with no response, and then calling back and being directed and redirected often times to non-English speakers. Dialing. Dead ends. Redialing. I was trying to move forward all while reeling in the constant disbelief that the snowbirds said the government wasn't going to do anything to help.

Kim had contacted other people and through the network of family and friends back home, in particular a close friend whose daughter somehow had connections through a friend of a friend with the US Embassy, I eventually received a call from an English-speaking woman with the US Consulate in Nuevo Vallarta. It turns out I should have been talking to the local consulate all morning instead of the embassy headquarters, but we didn't know that. The woman was an angel and she said they appointed a man with the consulate to be our 'go to' in helping us. I started to feel relief that things were finally moving forward in the search. Later that day, the consulate representative from Nuevo Vallarta visited us at the bungalow. Through his connections with local volunteer firefighters and other volunteers consisting of natives and snowbirds, tents had been set up next to our bungalow as a base camp for communication, and for organizing others to help with walking the beach and getting paddle boarders in the water. But that was it. Even with the consulate involved there were still no rescue boats, and no airplanes or helicopters. It was insane.

Kim had contacted her niece at KSTP-TV back home and they became instantly interested in our desperate situation in searching for Mark, and reporters conducted a phone interview with me and aired it on the news. We were under the impression that both the media and local government officials back home were working diligently with the consulate in Mexico, urging them to do what would routinely happen in the United States with Navy and Coast Guard involvement, with ships and smaller boats with divers below in the water and search airplanes and helicopters above, but in reality, there was nothing like that happening.

I was on autopilot from that moment on. Emotions went away. I wasn't weeping or feeling sorry for myself. I was enraged and distraught. I needed to stay focused and get the job done. I was so damn mad believing Mark was alive yet caught simultaneously in a state of complete desperation. I moved along in a robotic, mechanical fight mode. I had no time or energy for breaking down or crying.

While all the phone calling and organizing that was happening during the morning, what I did *not* know, as a result of my phone call home the night before to tell of Mark's disappearance, was that my brother Dave, and his wife Patti, had booked a flight for that morning and had arrived in Sayulita around noon trying to find me.

The moment Dave and Patti heard about Mark's disappearance they knew they needed to be there with me. There was no permission asked. No announcement was made. They needed to go, and they were going to go. I had no idea they were coming.

I sat hunched over outside on a bench in the common area of the bungalow. With all energy depleted I stared down a pathway. My distance vision is not good, and as I looked down the pathway, I saw something familiar. I looked more closely. Not something, but someone, *two* someone's, *Oh my god, it's Dave and Patti!* I called to them and they ran to me and we hugged tightly. With my mind and body spiraling in all kinds of emotions, I collapsed in their arms and sobbed with an intensity like never before. Dave and I are very close and I experienced and overwhelming sense of comfort that he and Patti were there with me, Kirk, and Liz, and I thought, *Good, everything is going to be okay now that they are here. Now we can move forward, we're not alone, and we're going to find Mark.*

Dave and Patti explained how they had found me, and that the minute I called them saying Mark was missing, they couldn't believe it was true, and that they were confident they would be able to find him. I looked at them perplexed as I didn't remember calling them, just as I had not remembered calling my friend Kim the night before either.

Dave and Patti had never been to Mexico and didn't know what to expect. Not of the sweltering heat or the rudimentary culture. They each had only a small backpack of clothes, and Dave wore his typical attire of black jeans, black cowboy boots, and black leather cowboy hat with a coon tail. Patti had on more summery clothing. They didn't know that a shuttle would be the most comfortable and quickest mode of transportation from Puerto Vallarta, so Patti suggested taking a public bus which took twice as long as a shuttle ride—over two hours. It was an overly crowded bus with no air conditioning which made frequent stops along the way to pick up folks holding chickens and crying babies, and they were extremely relieved to have finally arrived in Sayulita. They had never experienced the type of rustic foreign culture in which they had catapulted themselves into and were uncertain as to how concerned they should be for their safety. Dave had been a den chief in the Boy Scouts for many years and Patti a den mother assisting him, and both had learned much about preparedness, adaptability, and survivability. The first thing Dave bought when they arrived in Sayulita was a folding blade knife for their protection in the event they needed it. They didn't feel threatened necessarily—just uncertain and cautious of their unfamiliar surroundings. Patti said they knew we were staying at the trailer park and asked around the village looking for English speakers to tell them how to find it, and that they searched the town for a map and finally acquired one. They found a local bi-lingual speaker who directed them toward the ocean and to go across the river to find the trailer park. Well, during the rainy season it was actually a wide river, but in the dry season, it's a little tiny dribble of water that you splash in to walk across—like a stream of water running down the pavement when washing your car. But the locals simply refer to it year-round as the river. So Dave and Patti wandered around looking for a wider river as they finally made their way to the beach, and with the map, eventually found the trailer park.

Kirk had never met Dave, and upon observing him dressed in obvious non-beach attire of black jeans, black cowboy boots, black cowboy hat with a coon tail hanging from it, and the knife he had just bought attached to his belt, he pulled me aside asking, "Do I need to know anything about him? And do I need to worry about him?"

I looked at him with questioning eyes and said, "Are you kidding me? That's my brother. No, you don't need to worry about him. He dresses like that all the time."

Dave does present himself as a bit intimidating, but he is a softy inside. Both he and Patti are humble and benevolent toward others living their best according to one of the Boy Scout laws "to help other people at all times." They started dating in high school and got married when I was fifteen, and in 2013 had been married for 33 years, so Patti is more like a sister to me. They are a solid, beautiful, committed couple. They both ride Harley's, and before moving to Minneapolis after living in Colorado for about twenty years, Dave and his sons often went survivalist camping sleeping outside under the stars, and with those and other scouting skills they were prepared for the search.

With Kirk's concerns eliminated about Dave, we told Dave and Patti what happened with Mark's disappearance because they had very little second-hand information from my call home.

We decided they were going to stay with us and hunker down with me on the main level. It didn't matter that the space was small with only one bed. We were going to manage. And things were going to be okay.

Once Dave and Patti had more details about what had happened, they went searching for Mark. Their entire mindset was to find Mark that day, and then fly back home the next day. I wanted to help in the search somehow, but I was incapacitated inside the bungalow—debilitated while Dave and Patti searched fervidly for Mark, and Kirk and Liz manned the base camp tents beside the bungalow. Kirk and Liz remained the contacts for the volunteers handing out bottles of water and snacks for their periodic breaks, and to report if they had seen any sign of Mark. I paced inside the bungalow and at one point peered out the window watching as the paddle boarders looked only downward at the water waiting for the moment when they might see my Mark. I felt sick to my core. I moved away from the window so I could not see them any longer.

Other than making and taking phone calls to get the help we needed that morning, I spent the rest of the day moving from sitting tattered in the chair to roaming around inside the bungalow. Kirk and Liz forced me to sip water and to eat something, even just some crackers, both of which made me want to vomit. They encouraged me to sit outside in the common area to get some fresh air. I could not look at the water, and I did not go outside. How could I take any pleasure in sitting outside in that corner of paradise? Just breathing the fresh tropical air and listening to the birds chirping with the palm leaves rustling in the wind from inside the bungalow brought *horrible* guilt. Knowing Mark was out there either struggling for his life in the water or beached somewhere waiting for us, crushed me. I only felt okay staying in the one-room bungalow thinking I would have been better coiled in a dark closet denying myself of any pleasure. My stomach twisted tight and my head in a fog, I thought, *How can this be? How is this happening?* I wished I could erase the sights and stifle the sounds that taunted and tormented me to my core.

From the moment of Mark's disappearance, I remained at the bungalow. I did not go into the village. Anybody who was going to be doing anything to help find Mark had to come to me because I was going nowhere.

The daytime hours dragged painfully by until sundown when the base camp shut down with no news of finding Mark, and Dave and Patti returned disheartened and worn-out after searching and seeing no sign of him either. Dave said the expectation whenever they walked around a cove is that they would see Mark washed up wounded and waiting for help because it had not been that long since he went missing. And they did so with expectancy coupled with fear unsure of what they might find. They searched in detail, eyeing the surrounding area with a fine-toothed comb using walking sticks to poke in and around rock crevices and plants. They climbed cliffs to search the water from above with binoculars—all without success in finding Mark.

While Kirk, Liz, Dave, and Patti sat outside in the common area, I remained confined inside the bungalow unable to talk to anyone. Besides listening to the waves, I heard whispering amongst the four of them. I could not decipher their words, but I found solace in their quiet voices knowing they were near.

When it came time to go to sleep, Patti and I shared the bed while Dave slept on the cement bench in the open air outside the bungalow. I dozed off here and there, but I mainly just laid there thinking. Thinking and praying. Thinking about the present hellish situation. Thinking about the past. Praying for Mark to be found or for him to make his way to the bungalow.

I had been in a state of utter turmoil and disbelief at what was, and more importantly, what *was not* happening with the search effort. I thought about my children and could not imagine what it must be like for them to have received my dreadful phone call on that cold Minnesota winter night—now also in their own turmoil waiting for news about their dad.

I thought about Mark's siblings and the rest of my family back home, including my mom who had entered the middle stage of Alzheimer's. Thankfully, my sister Joanne was living with her and caring for her.

Kim had told me earlier that day that family, friends, and the community had come to our house to be with my Jacob, my Lucas, and my Sami.

As I laid distressed and sleepless in bed, I felt grateful for all that Kim was doing to get us the help we needed to find Mark. She and her husband, Joe, are dear friends.

Kim and Joe became good friends of ours starting in 1997 when they were still dating. We met them at a volleyball party at a mutual friend's house. Joe and I were playing volleyball on opposite teams, and Kim and Mark were on the sidelines watching. Kim noticed Mark sitting in a straight-back wooden chair. Not an outdoor lawn chair like everyone else sat in, but a kitchen chair that the hosts had let him use. Kim thought that was odd, so she asked him the reason for the wooden chair. Mark told her that he had recently undergone back surgery and needed to sit in an upright chair. The two of them hit it off right away and after the game the four of us chatted for a while, and we left the party without exchanging contact information. A few weeks later, we ran into them at a restaurant and soon afterward Kim and I grew close as I helped her with her hip issue as she trained in our home gym, and Mark and Joe became golf buddies and worked out together three days a week in our home gym as well. When Mark and Joe and their other friends went on golf trips, Mark used to tell me, with a wink and a sassy smirk, "Well, these don't really count as vacations. It's golf school!"

After my workouts with Kim, Mark often chimed in on our conversations when we came upstairs to the kitchen, and one time he offered to cook something for her knowing she must be hungry after the workout. She told him sure, so Mark pulled out a frozen chicken breast and put it in the microwave. That was his idea of cooking simply, and Mark didn't cook for anyone, so that was pretty fancy and special.

A few years after they were married, Joe and Kim had a baby girl, Maddie, and Mark and I were honored to be her godparents. Mark typically didn't take hold of other people's children, especially a newborn, but at Kim and Joe's first outing with Maddie, Mark was so proud to be her godfather that he immediately gravitated to her and his face beamed as he held and fed her.

As time moved on, Kim and I had become business partners in a women-only fitness club called, It Figures, that opened in 2002. It was initially Kim who urged me to get a club of my own. I was hesitant at first about the idea, but with Kim's tireless imploring to partner with me and the brainstorming sessions we had, we began to visualize what the club would look like. Sami, our youngest, was eight years old and in third grade and the timing seemed right. Kim said that my talent as a trainer, and the encouraging atmosphere I'd created in my home gym needed to be experienced by more women than just the few I trained there.

And she was right. The beautiful thing about the training sessions in our home gym was that as the women entered my house and walked into the kitchen before going downstairs to the gym, I ensured they felt welcomed by creating a warm and inviting atmosphere with flowers, coffee, tea, water, and fruit. I always asked how they were doing that day. Often-times we wouldn't make it past the kitchen island as unleashed emotions detailing how they were *really* doing that day came pouring out. They became comfort sessions, and it was okay if we didn't do a workout because what transpired during those sessions was as valuable and necessary as what was going to happen in the gym. For them and me. The camaraderie that I would have otherwise experienced out in the workforce I found in my own home. But even better.

Mark and I met with Kim and her husband, Joe, to discuss our idea about opening a club. The guys loved the idea, and we all agreed we'd finance the club together with Kim and I running the day-to-day operations.

When Kim and I went looking for space we found an available spot just a couple of blocks from our home. When we peered in through the window of the empty interior, we envisioned the club and where the equipment would be as well as its gathering place. We turned to one another and said, "This is it!"

We discussed where the counter should be, the one to replace my kitchen island, and that it should be at the front of the gym with the equipment toward the back.

At the time we opened It Figures, there was another national women-only franchise chain booming across the country. However, ours was quite different in that it wasn't only a place to get fit. It synthesized into something beyond our expectations. While we envisioned it to be a warm and inviting place, similar to our home gym, by creating a living room type atmosphere in the front area with fresh flowers, fruit, and beverages, we didn't foresee the birthing of a greater community of women that would ensue. I developed deeper relationships with women I'd only casually known from church, our children's school, and around town at various social gatherings as a result of opening the club. A community that would prove priceless to me in the years ahead.

We marketed our club as a wellness facility. The goal of our training was not only about exercising to lose weight, to tighten butts, and strive for six-pack abs, but to aim toward a healthy balance of body, mind, and spirit—full circle wellness. I consistently used, and still use, the phrase *tall, proud, posture* in the training sessions for inspiration. We focused on empowerment—to work from the inside out and the rest would take care of itself. We were about changing the motivation for exercise. A registered dietician was a member of the club, and she led nutritional presentations on a regular basis for the women. We had t-shirts created for the club that read WOW standing for Women Of Wellness, and it became a beautiful group of women supporting one another. It was also healthy for Sami to experience the kinship of women at such an early age, and Mark loved the direction we had taken.

The club was open Monday through Saturday, and during the week most of the women worked out before going to work, or back home as stay-at-home moms. Saturdays were a little different. We called it Bootcamp Saturday. It wasn't only another day for women to work out, but many stayed afterward to socialize because they didn't have to rush off anywhere, and those sessions typically lasted a couple of hours or more—cherished times for me and the others in so many different ways.

Kim and I opened the club on June 1, 2002, with a well-attended grand opening celebration that included family, friends, existing club members from my home gym, the local business and government community; along with new club members joining excited for a locally owned women's club. Mark's parents and my parents attended the opening, and they were all proud of our new venture. Mark's mom, Sena, gave me an intricate metal wire angel candle holder as a gift intended to be the guardian angel over the club, and I placed it in a special spot.

Unfortunately, the joy and excitement of opening the club was quickly met with heartbreak six days later when Mark's mom suddenly died at age seventy-nine as a result of a sepsis infection from a recent routine surgery she had undergone. His dad, Bill, a WWII Army veteran with a Purple Heart Medal for war wounds, and a Bronze Star Medal for bravery, sadly died three years later at age seventy-eight.

My father, John "Jack," had also served in the military in the Air Force during the Korean Conflict and had sadly passed away six years after we opened the club. His long-time condition of diabetes had worsened. It was good he and my mom lived nearby as I had the freedom to come and go from the club so that I could bring him to his appointments. Those times together were precious—a gift. He ended up in the emergency room where he eventually passed away surrounded by our family. And a favorite memory I have during my dad's last hours is sharing his favorite candy with him. Bit-O-Honey. My mom was still alive, and I felt honored to have her as a card-carrying member of the club.

Mark and I each had close relationships with our parents while growing up and those relationships carried on into our marriage and with our children.

Mark and his dad shared a love of sports and history, and he adored his mother who had been a homemaker, and also worked for the phone company. He was her *Marky* and raising him had been effortless for them.

I was a tomboy growing up and shared a love of sports with my dad also. He took me under his wing as he coached me in many sports, and he lovingly called me his *Nanny*. And I admired my loving mom who worked selflessly to help provide for me and my five siblings as a homemaker.

When I moved to Minneapolis at age nineteen, I felt torn between living near my parents in a small town and loving the city life. But then fifteen years later, when Jacob, Lucas, and Sami were young my parents moved to Minneapolis and bought a house about a mile away from us. We were blessed to have them close by and saw them often along with Mark's parents. The social life for both sets of parents was family, and Mark and I often reflected on how fortunate we were to have wonderful parents and our children's grandparents involved in our lives.

We owned the club for nine years and sold it in 2011. It Figures had been a success on so many levels. Not from a financial standpoint in the end, but a successfully important place for hundreds of women over the years of whom many are now my life-time friends, and for whom many possess their own friendships they might not otherwise have developed.

Though the club doors had closed many women continued working out in our home gym. Just a handful of women worked out during the week, and anywhere from ten to fifteen women continued showing up for Bootcamp Saturday offering us the luxury of time, and I occasionally included bloody marys and mimosas into the mix. In the winter we hung out in my kitchen, and on the warmer days we lounged on our secluded garden patio. The wonderful community of It Figures, is why, when Mark went missing, that my friends from the club and the community wrapped its arms around our family and our home in Robbinsdale.

Robbinsdale has been recently nicknamed Birdtown after its close spelling to the bird, and not after the man, Robbins, who founded the city. It's only three-square miles with a population of about 14,000 people. The people at our house with our children while we were in Mexico I had christened, Team Birdtown, because it included not only family and friends, but also fellow commissioners, council members, the mayor, parishioners, local business owners and other people I personally did not know who reached out to my family—a community that came together to embrace and uphold us within the calamity. "Only in Birdtown." It's a common phrase I use with my family and friends to say how wonderful it is to live in Robbinsdale. It seems normal for folks who live in small towns to come together in support of their fellow residents, but Robbinsdale borders the city of Minneapolis with nearly half a million people, so we're really just an extension of the larger city. But Birdtown is special. It has a small-town feel and is a vibrant community with unique shops and restaurants operated by small business owners.

I found comfort knowing my children were surrounded by loving close family and friends to feed them, to hold them, to cry with them, to hope and pray with them, and to just *be* with them while I was over 2,000 miles away. My children had my family and Team Birdtown with them, and I had Team Sayulita with me.

Kim and another friend of ours, Tom, had started a CaringBridge page on the first day of the search-and-rescue to keep people informed of developments. The post stated that when Mark and I were on vacation in Sayulita, Mark had been pulled out to sea by a riptide and that I watched helplessly from the beach as he was pulled further and further from the shore, and that he has not been seen since. The post went on to say that Mark is a father of three children with much to live for, and that all who know him realize he is a strong and determined man who could survive this situation, and that everyone is hoping he will soon be found safe. Tom had also spent hours in contact with the Minnesota State Senate office to see about coordinating the two countries search effort. His attempt proved unsuccessful for reasons having to do with international treaties preventing a joint effort.

I need to add a disclaimer. It is clear from the beginning of Mark's disappearance that some wrong information had been passed along. It was not the riptide that caused Mark to vanish, but the giant white-water waves that crashed down upon him. There was so much mayhem with phone calling and texting and dealing with the Mexican government, the embassy and consulate, and local volunteers, that information had not always circulated correctly. Nothing about the task at hand was tidy and straightforward.

I was thankful my sister-in-law, Tina, took over my Facebook page as an additional place to keep people informed of developments. There was no way I had the mental well-being or interest to update Facebook. My interest existed in the sole mission to find Mark.

Sami texted me again throughout the night. *Hi, mom. How are you doing? I love you.* We had texted each other throughout the day as well. I really don't know of any in-depth conversations with her. I'm sure I heard her voice. I'm sure we talked. Why wouldn't we? I remember the middle of the night texting more than anything because talking was such a struggle, and with Patti lying next to me I didn't want to bother her. We didn't need to text many words. We were simply there for each other.

Besides the necessary texting and phone calling with Kim to get the processes moving with the embassy and the consulate, interviews with the media back home and treasured texting with Sami, I didn't text much, except for check-ins with Jacob, Lucas, and my sister Joanne. I really don't like texting. I'd rather talk, but I had no emotional wherewithal to do so. It felt like my mouth was on mute except for the interviews with news channels and newspapers. I was more than willing to talk to the media to raise awareness in order to move forward with the search-and-rescue. Then I could do my job. But just talking with people wasn't doing my job. It wouldn't have served any purpose except to try to make me feel better, and I did not want to feel better.

I would've felt guilty having an open conversation with someone afraid that it might turn into talking about niceties like the weather. There were no niceties to discuss. I needed to talk to people who were going to get the information out and expand the search for my Mark.

This was the second sleepless night I spent clutching Mark's shorts to my chest. The constant pounding of the waves racked my nerves. I silently cussed at them; inwardly screamed at them. A sea of unappeasable fury. I couldn't stop my mind from seeing him out there and wondering, *Was that the wave that brought him ashore?*

ELEVEN

Day 6—Second Day Of Search, Thursday, February 28th

The sun rose and the birds chirped as if it were just another day in paradise. But for us it was everything but that.

It had been a restless night for all five of us. Dave said that as he laid on the cement bench, he could feel Mark's presence as he listened to the raucous ocean while remaining hypervigilant about every sound around. He expected Mark to walk up at any moment seeing him lying there and gruffly demanding, "What are *you* doing here? You were worried about me? Why? I knew I was going to be okay—I'm Mark!"

Dave and Patti headed out at dawn for their second day of searching equipped again with their walking sticks, binoculars, and folding knife. Dave again wore his jeans, cowboy boots, and cowboy hat, but instead of wearing his long sleeve button-down shirt, he wore a black t-shirt that he bought in town and cut off the sleeves. Patti again wore more summery clothes and sturdy tennis shoes. Their first day they searched the northside of the beach where Mark disappeared, just like I'd done the first night, but planned to search the southside since the locals said that is the direction the waves move.

While Dave and Patti were out searching, Kirk and Liz again manned the base camp, and I, again, remained anguishing inside the bungalow primarily in the fetal position on the chair or in the bed—writhing in anxiousness with no appetite and ceaselessly begged God for Mark's return.

On this same day, another CaringBridge post unintentionally reported incorrect information stating that due to the media and pressure from the US government, that Mexican Navy helicopters and boats were searching, and that the embassy was involved. The post closed requesting prayers for a successful rescue.

Again, I need to add a disclaimer. As far as I knew, there were no Mexican Navy helicopters in the air or boats in the water, as we likely would have seen them from the shore. We were told there was some Navy awareness, but we never saw activity, and it was the consulate, not the embassy assisting us. Also, the search parties on the ground were not government officials. From our understanding they consisted of Dave and

Patti, local volunteer firefighters, and other volunteers. At one point, I peeked out at the beach and saw a man flying a drone over the land and water, and again painfully watched paddle boarders scouring the waters below them to see if Mark was still in the area.

Earlier that morning, I spoke to a newspaper reporter from back home and he published an article that same day, with the headline, again, well-intentioned but incorrect, reporting that a riptide had taken Mark out to sea while body surfing. Yes, a riptide took him out, but that's not what caused him to vanish. The headline was correct, however, in reporting that I watched in horror, and the article included a photo of Mark and I in Florida just a few weeks earlier in January.

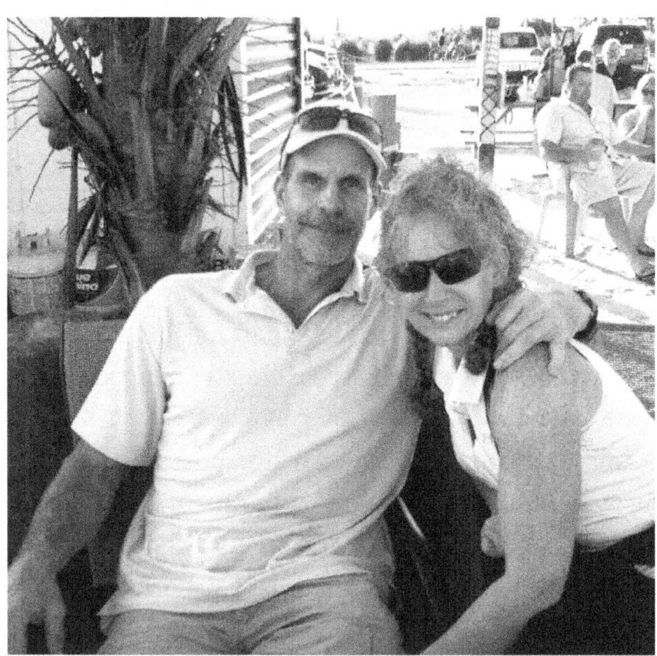

Mark and I in Florida-January 2013

The news story continued stating that Mark was fifty-eight years old and a near forty-year lineman for Xcel Energy ready to retire. He mentioned our three grown children, and that Mark and I were on a winter getaway for our 26th wedding anniversary vacationing in Sayulita, while expounding on the fact we'd been to Mexico many times before. In the article I was reported as saying it was just insane. I explained that as it got dark, the local authorities said we had to wait until morning, and that other locals said it will take a few days and the body will wash to shore. It was like a dog had drowned. He reported divers were out again Thursday morning, and we were waiting for more teams from Puerto Vallarta, and that searchers have also been scouring the beaches.

Another disclaimer. It may have been that we were told there was going to be divers in the water. Or that is what I thought would be the case as that is typical protocol in the United States, but there were never any divers. And…we were *not* in the United States.

The reporter was genuinely sympathetic during the interview. He continued to write that I believed Mark was stranded somewhere among the rocks and cliffs, or along the shoreline waiting for help. He wrote that I choked back my emotions as I told him about the moment Mark was swept away while in the water with Kirk.

I told the reporter that it had been a fabulous day. That the guys scooted out for a little bit of bodysurfing because the waves were perfect for it, that we could see the bigger waves coming in, and that right then was when we needed something, a board or something. I explained to the reporter that if Kirk had gone in after Mark in those treacherous conditions without a flotation device, it would have made the situation even worse. That then there may have been *two* people missing. I ended the interview saying I was staying in Mexico as long as I needed because, "I can't come home without him."

People might wonder why Mark and Kirk went into the water if the waves were so rough. When the four of us walked down the beach together, the waves had been a body surfers dream. Mark and Kirk entered the water with perfect waves, caught the first set, and rode in effortlessly. Then in an instant, things changed. It was a combination of the rip that suddenly pulled Mark out about fifty feet coupled with a set of rogue waves appearing out of nowhere. If the waves that hit Mark would have been the same size as those in the first set, Mark would have survived, and he would have known how to swim out of a rip. If I, or anyone, could have gone in to save him, we would have, but the thunderous waves made that impossible. Even with a flotation device, the rescue would have been extremely risky.

In the midst of all the turmoil and trauma, that same day Verizon informed me that I'd nearly reached the maximum allowable minutes on my plan, and that they were going to cut me off. *Are you kidding me! They are talking about cutting off my lifeline to family, friends, and people who were assisting in finding my Mark.* I'd pleaded with them to increase my minutes due to a life and death emergency. I explained the circumstances for the excessive phone calling and texting urging them to verify the reasons with media sources in Minneapolis and the US Consulate. Thankfully, Verizon confirmed the reasons why and extended my plan for as long as I needed it during the search-and-rescue.

Around mid-afternoon Dave and Patti returned to the bungalow after hours of trudging along the southern shore for three miles under the scorching sun. They wrestled through outcroppings of rocks and foraged through scrub brush intently inspecting every potential spot where Mark might be marooned. They sidestepped around rocks and waited for the incoming tide to roll out so they could quickly walk before it rolled back in again. They clambered up into the hills over rugged terrain hoping to see better with binoculars and back down again. They searched high and low until they reached a secured private resort and then had to turn back. They said they started to be concerned about their safety as they climbed up into the hills, and Dave said he wished he would have had a machete. Not only for chopping through the brush, but for their physical safety with the possibility of coming upon giant iguanas. They also wondered about their safety if found trespassing on land owned by a non-English speaker, and the owner then demanding to explain what they were doing there. Neither Dave nor Patti spoke Spanish except for a few basic words.

Dave told me he thought it would be really important for me to be able to see our children and for them to see me, as well as other family members and friends so I could update everyone on the status of the search. Dave had already connected with Kim and our friend, Tom, back home to coordinate a live feed from me in Mexico at a local bar and restaurant, The Eagle's

Nest Lounge, on their large screen the following night on Friday. He said it was being planned as a vigil.

When Dave told me about the plan, I felt comforted by the continual outpouring of love and support from him and Patti, Kirk and Liz, and everyone back home. I yearned so badly to be with my children and was excited to finally be able to see them even if only on video. Dave and Patti scouted around the bungalow premises asking if anyone had a computer with internet service. They found a lovely couple nearby more than willing to let us use theirs.

A while later, the consulate contacted me saying they needed copies of our passports and the location where we were staying. Dave and Patti walked into town to find a business with a fax machine. They found a place where they could fax it themselves, but the instructions were all in Spanish. They asked around and found an English speaker at a real estate office who would fax it for them, but the power in the entire town was down so they were told to come back hourly to see if the power was back up. It was another reminder that we were not in the USA. After a couple of walks back into town, Dave and Patti were finally able to fax the documents to the consulate.

After sunset, friends back home wrote another CaringBridge post informing people that Mark had not yet been found, that everyone continues to be hopeful, that they send well wishes to me and the search-and-rescue crew, and announced the candlelight vigil at 7 pm the next night at The Eagle's Nest Lounge.

It was another sleepless night despite how exhausted I was from a second full day of interviews, weariness from the anger and frustration that not enough was being done to find Mark, and worrying about my children back home.

I laid in bed hoping and praying for the best, but in my heart of hearts, began to fear for the worst. I had to continually force myself out of the fearful mindset and remain hopeful concerned that I might otherwise spiral out of control. I thought about what an amazing family life we had over the years. I thought about what a loving, giving, husband and father Mark had been through thick and thin. We had a special family bond.

I don't know how many families can say that their fifty-eight-year-old father plays softball on the same team as their early twenty-something sons. Mark, Jacob, and Lucas spent much time together whether at the house or out and about. Often-times teens and young adults go off on their own, but our situation was different. They wanted to be around us. Jacob bought his first house when he was twenty-one. Yet, for four years before Mark died, Jacob spent a lot of time with us hanging around wanting to be with the family. And I know there are a lot of young people who move out and say, "Okay bye, see you on the holidays!" But that's not our family style. Lucas and Sami still lived at home and they liked being at home with the family. Whether it was a BBQ or pot roast, or just everyday living, our house was the happiest when bursting at the seams with people.

In the earlier years, we didn't allow TVs in our children's bedrooms. If we watched TV, we did so together in the family room.

We had an open-door policy in our home, so much so that I had to be careful to shut my bedroom door when I was changing because there were people wandering in all the time whether it was the kid's friends, family, or our friends.

Over time we transformed our side yard into a fun place to play, relax, and eat. We installed a large hot tub when Jacob and Lucas were about four and two years old and made them wear little life jackets. About ten years later, we created a rolling putting green with artificial turf and planted trees and a variety of flowering plants to traverse the area. We had a huge gas grill and large table for gatherings. It was our retreat. And it brought people to us. The last thing Mark wanted to do on a Friday night after driving all week and working long hard hours, was to get in a car and drive to a cabin to do more work. So, we created our own haven at home.

Mark and I felt blessed that our children wanted to be at home with us. That was the greatest gift of all—the feeling of them wanting to be with us. As they grew older, we didn't have to get on the phone and beg our children to come over. If anything, it was almost the opposite with us telling them we think it's time to go home.

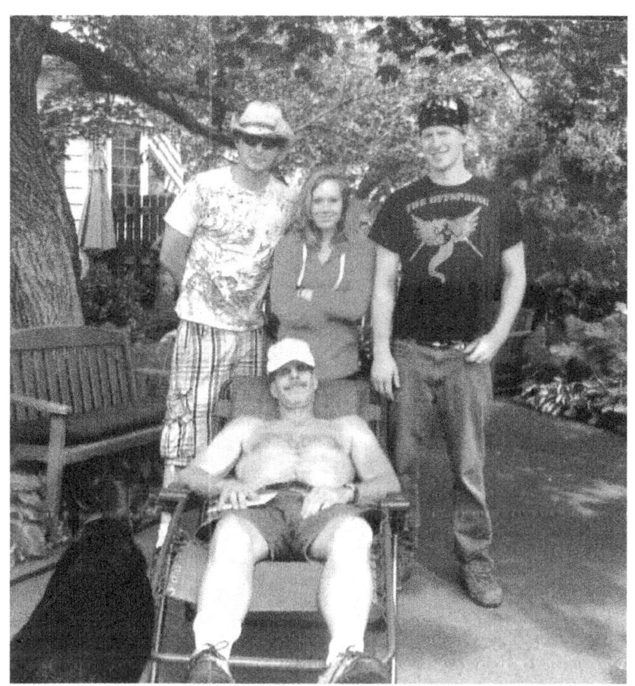

Jacob, Sami, Lucas, Mark, and dog Chaser-2012. Mark in his zero-gravity lounge chair as a Father's Day gift.

For the third night in a row, Sami's short middle of the night texts helped me get through the hours upon hours of listening to the pitiless tormenting torture of the surf.

I thought back to the time when Mark and Sami went shopping for boots for her 2012 summer job, only nine months before Mark's disappearance. Sami went away to the Minnesota Conservation Corp (MCC). It is a natural environmental camp teaching and empowering teenagers to be pro-actively engaged learners, while working jobs to manage natural resources in parks and public lands such as stream bank stabilization, trail construction, and invasive species management.

The MCC prohibited cell phone usage as a form of communication. In order for teens to communicate with their parents and others back home, they had to write letters. If there was a need for parents or teens to call one another, they notified the staff who in turn managed the respective requests according to program guidelines.

Before Sami left for the camp, Mark insisted that he bring her shopping for the boots she needed for the eight-week program. As a lineman he knew the importance of wearing high-quality work boots. He knew Sami was going to be laboring for long hours each day in all weather conditions working on various types of terrain with heavy lifting, digging, shoveling, and using heavy tools like chain saws and brush saws to fulfill the MCC mission of habitat restoration. Mark did *not* want her wearing trendy fashion boots or even standard hiking boots that others might be wearing. He bought her the kind of boots he wore as a lineman—durable enough to withstand constant wear and tear. The boots were waterproof, lightweight, and flexible with soles designed to move with her foot with slip resistant treads.

That shopping trip with just the two of them was meaningful on many levels. As with most teens who are coming into their own sense of identity apart from their parents, often thinking their parents don't know what they're talking about, or that they know better than mom and dad; whether she trusted him or not with the boot shopping, she went along with the idea.

It wasn't only about the boots. It was also about *that* specific shopping experience with just the two of them that was much bigger than a person might think. Mark shopping with our children never happened in our house. For all our married years I did the shopping. Whether it was clothes, birthday, or Christmas presents, grocery shopping for our family meals or the parties we had—that was my gig because I had the luxury of being home. I never expected him to do those things. Granted, if he wanted to, it would have been nice to have him involved in some of that shopping, but it didn't happen that way.

That shopping trip with Sami was significant for Mark. I think he may have been worried as to how he was going to deal with his baby girl being gone for eight weeks, and he needed to offer her something special.

It took her a few days before she realized dad knew what he was talking about, and thank goodness he did because she had an edge over many of the others. While many of the participants dealt with soggy, uncomfortable feet, Sami's boots turned out to be a game changer for her. She rocked it. Those boots were exactly what she needed, and in one of the letters she sent home she wrote how grateful she was that dad took her shopping. For Sami to put it into words on paper in a handwritten letter to her father thanking him was precious beyond anything. It was a pivotal moment in their relationship.

<p style="text-align:center">~~~~~~</p>

The daytime hours on Wednesday and Thursday had brought great hope. But as the daylight waned, hope waned too. Like a candle feebly fluttering and holding on to its last flicker until consumed by the liquid wax. It was that unavoidable. The daytime provided fresh new eyes. A feeling like, *this is going to be the day*. But the nighttime, every time it went dark all I wondered was, *Is Mark out there alive and stranded on a rock island or beach nearby, or in the ocean floating on debris, alone, cold and in the dark?* For Mark, I thought that daytime as well would have brought hope as he either waited to be found beached somewhere, or clinging onto something trying to make his way to shore. I dreaded what nighttime would have been doing to his mind, body, and soul. Out in the fading moonlit darkness hearing only the sound of the ceaseless, cruel, slapping of the waves as he laid injured on land or against whatever scrap of debris he clung onto for dear life. Once the darkness fell there became a sense of hopelessness and helplessness. Just a terrible feeling knowing there would be no rest. My mind reeled envisioning the moments that the tragedy happened, contrasted with flashes of bits and pieces of our lives together as husband and wife, and dad and mom. I was stuck from looking forward. There was an impenetrable dark wall that could not be broken through. Like drying concrete squeezing my brain. And the reason I couldn't get beyond it was because I'd never been there before. My forward imagination ceased. It was dreadful.

I yearned for the sound of the waves to silence themselves so I could maybe hear him calling for help. But there was such bad intention on the part of the savage sea. As with the other two nights there was no shred of solace from the torturous indifferent crush of the waves on my being. My mind was stuck in the muck and mire, like a seashell buried in the wet sand, and I continually wondered, *Was that the wave that brought him ashore?*

TWELVE

Day 7—Third Day Of Search, Friday, March 1st

Dave and Patti, just like the other days, left at dawn to search for Mark armed with walking sticks, a knife, and binoculars. The night before, they washed their few pieces of clothing they had packed—thinking they would be with us for one day—hung them to dry, and they were dry by morning. Kirk and Liz again faithfully manned the base camp tent providing water and snacks for the volunteer firefighters, and other volunteers in continuing the search effort with paddle boards in the water while others walked the beach.

My sister Joanne texted me that a local cable channel had been at our home on Thursday videotaping and interviewing my family. The reporters were in the studio reporting while segueing back and forth with the video footage in our home.

The two-minute video panned the kitchen counter piled high with food provided by family, friends, and the community, and showed my loved ones sitting at the kitchen table quietly chatting, hugging, and filled with hope.

They spoke individually to our daughter, Sami, and Joanne. Joanne was shown standing by a window responding to a question saying, "We just want to know. We just need information." And referring to the footage of the lineup of cars on the street in front of our house and the plentiful food on the countertop, Joanne said, "It means everything, and for me it shows me just how loved Mark and his family are."

The reporter in the studio said, "Family and friends must do the hardest thing of all."

My Sami is quoted saying, "He's one of the strongest, most healthy, well rounded men that you could probably ever meet. If anyone could live or float in the water, it would be him and we need him to come back. We're just waiting. There's nothing else we can do."

The reporter stated that search crews with the Mexican Navy were combing the sea and beaches for Mark, and they showed a photo of Mark on the screen provided by my family.

Again, another disclaimer. The only people combing the beaches were the volunteers. The Mexican Navy was not involved.

A recording of my voice from my cell phone played with a photo of me displayed on the screen, and I told the reporter, "I believe in miracles, so I'm hopeful. I have faith. My family has faith. And whatever the outcome is…well, you know, we'll accept it, but I won't give up until it's over."

They showed three more photos of Mark and me, and the reporter informed the TV audience that there was a CaringBridge page updating family and friends with the latest news on the search. The reporter said that with search boats in the water and helicopters in the air that there is hope that Mark, being a strong athletic lineman, would survive the powerful current that swept him out to sea.

Again, there were no boats, and no helicopters, and it was not the rip current that caused him to vanish.

I explained to the reporter, "The reason they are still somewhat considering it a search-and-rescue is that there's a chance my husband got beyond the break and taken by the current, and could be on one of many lock areas or abandoned beaches. It's no less important now than it was before—to keep the pressure on local and government authorities in Mexico to continue the search efforts."

The report ended with another photo of Mark, and then me saying I was working with a representative with the US Embassy, (it was actually the consulate), in Mexico, that I intended to keep the pressure on until Mark was found, and that there was going to be a vigil held that night with Father Bryan Pedersen of Sacred Heart Church in Robbinsdale leading the vigil.

Around midday, Dave and Patti returned to the bungalow. They used their map and walked about ten miles along the road above where they'd been the day before, to see if they could get beyond the private resort and back down to the water's edge on a peninsula. They had again been concerned for their safety, not only from locals who may have considered them as trespassers, but also from trucks, busses, and cars speeding by them as they skirted close to the brush on the winding shoulderless narrow highway. At one point in their trek, they ended up having to jump into a ditch when they saw an oncoming car driving too close to them. It took them about five hours to walk ten miles in the blistering heat until they reached the private resort. They approached a staff person at the resort gate entrance asking if they would let them walk through their property to the ocean to search for their brother-in-law who had gone missing in the water. The staff member spoke English and said, "No." They asked for water, but the staff member wouldn't give them any. They both realized they had walked way beyond where they should have, but their goal was to find Mark. Dave's feet bled inside his boots and Patti sat down on the ground exhausted, crying, and saying she couldn't walk anymore. Dave then asked the staff member to please call a taxi for them as his cell phone was dead. He agreed and called a taxi. Their grueling five-hour walk had only been a twenty-minute drive back to the village.

A short while later, a man approached the base camp saying he had been vacationing in Puerto Vallarta when he read about Mark's disappearance in the local newspaper. His name was David, and he said he had previously conducted international search-and-rescue efforts as a pilot, and that he had connected with someone he knew at the National Oceanic and Atmospheric Administration (NOAA) about Mark's disappearance, and that they had a pretty good idea which direction Mark would have been taken out to sea because of the tides and currents on that day.

I was inside the bungalow when Dave, Patti, Kirk, and Liz came to me telling me about the pilot and to come outside. As I listened to him and heard what he had to say, hope arose within me, and I felt he was nothing less than an angel falling from heaven. I know the others felt the same way. I thought, *What are the odds that an international search-and-rescue pilot, I believe from Canada, happened to be on vacation an hour south and read in the newspaper about Mark, and deemed it necessary to come and find us.* It was an amazing turn of events.

NOAA uses real-time data collected from their Search And Rescue Satellite Aided Tracking (SARSAT) satellites for both sea and land operations. The satellites determine the speed and direction of tides and currents, and monitors weather conditions at any given time throughout the day all over the world. Tides start in the ocean and rise and fall as they push toward the shore, while currents simultaneously move the water back and forth.

David graciously offered his time to fly an airplane over the coast to search for Mark, and that with his expertise and the SARSAT data he could narrow the search area to about three hundred square miles. David told us on the day that Mark disappeared the current was different than normal. He said typically the current flowed in one direction outward in the 'river of garbage,' however, on that day, after he reviewed the satellite data, he discovered there were three currents flowing—one straight out, one to the left, and another to the right. It's called a river of garbage because of how the current grabs the waves on either side of itself, including sand, debris, and natural sea life, and quickly and forcefully funnels it all outward from the shore.

He encouraged us saying he believed Mark could still be alive on a beach somewhere on one of the many small uninhabited rocky islands, or holding onto something adrift in the water like a barrel or a log, as it was not uncommon to have all types of debris floating in the water, and said he could obtain a search-and-rescue airplane out of Puerto Vallarta the next morning. The five of us were astounded and profoundly humbled by his offer.

We contacted the consulate representative and asked if there were plans for any airplanes or helicopters from the Mexican government, and we were told, "No."

"What do you think about *us* putting an airplane in the air?" I asked.

The representative said, "We do not recommend it."

I then told David the pilot to move ahead with the airplane and agreed that since he was volunteering his time, I would pay for the airplane and fuel with the cash that Mark had stashed around the bungalow on our first day in Sayulita. I did not tell the consulate representative that we were moving ahead on our own. I imagine the reason the consulate, and maybe even the embassy, didn't want us to hire our own pilot is that it would look like they weren't doing enough—that now these tourists from the USA have to pay for their own search effort and it wouldn't look good for them—especially with the media.

WCCO News, another local news source back home contacted me that day, and when I told them about David the pilot, they quoted me saying, "The man is 'an angel' and that he works all over the world and has contacts you wouldn't imagine." The reporter stated that I said a Mexican Navy rescue team was also assisting in the search effort. As I have previously stated, that simply was not the case as far as we were aware.

I then thought about the upcoming video conference that evening with my children and everyone back home at the restaurant, and became anxious. As time grew closer, Dave, Patti, Kirk, and Liz made sure I took time to at least present myself well, not needing to primp too much, but to at least make myself look decent in front of the camera. I didn't necessarily want to look good; I just didn't want to look bad. The last thing I wanted was for our children to see me strung out and on deaths door having secluded myself in the bungalow the past four nights and three days. I was nervous about how I'd sound—hopefully without a shaky voice. I wanted to be strong and confident. And that was so difficult to think about doing because so much of my time until then had been spent saying little, doing little, and curled into myself and inside my own thoughts. To have to speak was going to take a major effort. To know that our children were going to be out there looking at me and wondering what they needed to see—it was a big deal. It was their only opportunity to see me, and it was important that I display strength.

Around 6:30 pm the five of us gathered two doors down at the couple's trailer who had the computer for the live video feed. I took time to steady myself. At 7 pm we went live. A huge crowd had gathered in support of our family. To be looking at my Jacob, my Lucas, and my Sami on the screen along with the crowd of family and friends was overwhelming. But I had to keep it together. I had to stay strong. I looked intently into the computer screen and said, "Make no mistake. When that airplane goes out tomorrow, know that this is not a search-and-recovery effort. It is a search-and-rescue. The pilot and all of us believe there is a very good chance Mark is alive holding onto something, or on the shore somewhere nearby." And everyone back home cheered.

The video conference lasted only a few minutes, but it had a monumental impact. My resolve to continue pressuring the consulate and the Mexican government to increase the search effort further intensified, but mentally and physically preparing for the live feed and seeing my children and so many other family and friends further consumed me. Afterward, I walked straight back to the bungalow and again nestled myself inside the Mexican blanket and clutched Mark's shorts as my pillow.

Friday night brought with it continued sleeplessness in anticipation of the Saturday morning sunrise at 7:30 when David, in his bubble front search airplane, would be flying over the waters of Sayulita looking for Mark.

Sami again, for the fourth night in a row faithfully texted asking how I was doing, what I was thinking, and we always ended with, "I love you."

Even though hope had been revived with plans for the search airplane in the morning, I experienced another long struggle to keep sane with the waves continually thrashing on the shore. When my nerves seemed near the breaking point, I prayed for strength to withstand the merciless provoking of the waves creating a constant friction inside my brain. Strength, *tangible* strength eluded me. The very ocean that soothed our souls the first three nights of our trip, became a repressive dictator whose unjust authority exasperated me into a crumpled heap of near nothingness. I could only wonder, *Was that the wave that brought him ashore?*

THIRTEEN

Day 8—Fourth Day Of Search, Saturday, March 2ⁿᵈ

At daybreak, the five of us went outside the bungalow and surely enough, within a few minutes, we heard an airplane engine. *Oh, my god.* It was the craziest thing. We knew we were breaking a rule—the consulate recommended not to do it, yet there we were hunkering down wide-eyed waiting for the airplane to appear.

The five of us threw out questions to each other. Questions with no known answers.

"What *are* the rules? Will we get into trouble with the Mexican government? The US government? What if they shoot him down!" Until then, we had not considered any possible ramifications. We just thought, *Damn it! We don't care. We're doing it!*

When the airplane came into view it was breathtaking. Ethereal. It was as though David the pilot was our Superman coming to the rescue to find Mark. We had an incredible, euphoric feeling that *finally* more was being done after so many other hours upon hours and days with little being done—except for volunteers. We all felt like we were being so bad and yet so good.

David flew over and greeted us with a tipped wing as if saying, *I've got this*, and then flew out over the ocean. We lost sight of him after a while as he planned to weave back and forth twenty miles out to sea and fifteen miles south paralleling the land. It was so very troubling to see him need to fly out that far. I was so sure he was going to find Mark, but wavered within a convoluted cluster of emotions as to the condition in which he would be found.

I went back to the bungalow. Kirk and Liz stayed at the base camp, and Dave and Patti went back out searching to the south because that was where David the pilot was flying. The volunteers were out again walking the beach with the paddle boarders again searching downward into the waters.

Meanwhile, back home, Kim updated the CaringBridge site saying she spoke with me today and that I was overwhelmed with seeing and receiving the kindness of so many people back home at The Eagle's Nest Lounge vigil. Kim also thanked everyone who donated money at the vigil for whatever we may need as a family, and for people to keep praying for our family and the continued search-and-rescue. She informed everyone that David the NOAA pilot was going to search that day. I don't know if David was a NOAA pilot or if he used the NOAA data for his search effort, but people back home referred to him as the NOAA pilot.

I was unaware that there was going to be a request for donations at the vigil, and I had warmth in my heart for all who were there and for their generosity in giving.

The donations had been organized by a dear friend of ours who was collecting the money to fly Jacob, Lucas, and Sami to Sayulita to be with me while we searched for Mark. When Kim called me that next morning and told me of the plan, I told her I was grateful for the good-willed intention thinking it would be best if my children were with me, but I told her no and the reasons why and she understood. The last thing I needed was for my children to be with me, not because I didn't want them there, but more than anything it wouldn't have been safe for them; and emotionally I had nothing to offer in the way of comforting them. I wasn't sleeping and not doing well at all. I explained that we were in a tiny bungalow and there would be no place for them to sleep, and that Dave had to sleep on the cement bench outside. Sure, we could have obtained additional housing, but for me to be worried about my children in a place that has dangerous waters and concerned something might happen to them if they went looking for their dad; and not knowing when or if their dad might be found severely injured on a nearby beach, I thought the last place they needed to be was with me and the others. It would *not* have been good. Not good at all. They needed to be safe at home with my family and friends.

About midmorning, I met via cell phone with five friends who I'd grown close to through the It Figures bootcamp. They weren't at my home where they'd been with our children the last few days, but instead at a local bakery, and we sat on speaker phone with each other. They were so sweet and concerned, and felt the need for me to describe my environment so they could have more of a connection with me. They wanted to know what the bungalow looked like, so I took photos and sent them to them. I clutched the Mexican blanket, my *security blanket*, that I bought the day Mark went missing and set it on the various places I had been around the bungalow. Three places to be exact. On the bed, on the chair, and on the cement bench. That was the first time, with the exception of Kim, that I'd spoken at length to friends back home since Mark's disappearance. I cherished that time with them but had little to offer in my depleted state of existence. Though my hope had been regenerated with David the pilot searching for Mark, and his confidence that Mark might be hanging onto debris in the ocean, or stranded on one of the many rock islands, I'd become mentally and physically tapped out. I had been enduring through hope. Unquantifiable hope. Simply hoping and envisioning that David would find Mark uplifted my soul. But I still had nothing to offer to anyone.

Later that morning, one of my friends in that group called me back. I must have sounded very down and vulnerable in the group conversation, and as a result, in a voice of confidence my friend said, "Nancy, you've got this."

Those four little words deeply impacted me. She knew it was something I needed to hear. It was one of the most powerful things that I heard because I could hear it in her voice that she believed in me. It wasn't a cheerleader type of you've got this. It was more like, no matter what happens, you've got this. And I believed her. I needed to believe her. She believed in me even when I struggled to believe in myself. No one in my life ever needed to say that to me before. It was empowering, definitely necessary, and so instrumental for me moving forward to the next...*whatever.*

A little while later I called Jacob. Since the night that Mark went missing, I had communicated with him only through short texts but primarily through texts with Sami on his and Lucas's behalf. Other than that, I hadn't actually spoken to him. All three of our children had been experiencing devastating heartache despite the love of concerned people surrounding them, and I knew they were all handling their immeasurable anguish in different ways. I wanted to encourage him so he could in turn encourage Lucas and Sami with the hope that the rescue pilot knew where to look for their dad. The conversation became instantly electrified when we heard each other's voices. He heard the sound of confidence in my voice, and 2,000 miles away I heard his voice rise up strong, and I envisioned him standing tall and proud. He said he would take care of things and for me not to worry about them back home, and that I needed to stay focused on finding their dad.

David the pilot told us he planned to search for three to four hours. We tried to estimate when he would return to Sayulita after conducting the search; landing in Puerto Vallarta, then driving back up to us, and figured he'd arrive around 2:30 pm.

We started to grow anxious an hour after his expected time of arrival. No David. Two more hours went by. No David. Two and a half hours and still no David. It was only an hour drive. *Where are you, David?*

Finally, I don't know who saw him first, but David came walking into the bungalow area, and I didn't know what to think or feel. I thought, *I don't know what I want to hear.* My head spun thinking of so many scenarios. I thought maybe he was going to tell us that he didn't spot Mark. If that were the case, then there was still hope. But he could have also been coming to tell us that he *did* find him, but if *that* were the case, he likely would have called me. And then I thought if Mark was found lifeless, then David would have wanted to tell us in person. My emotions began to churn to the surface ready to explode like from inside a volcano.

David approached us with a hesitant tight-lipped half grin carrying a long roll of paper—it was a map. He suggested we find a place where we could all view the map, so he and the five of us walked to the restaurant next to the bungalow. I studied his body language and demeanor as we walked, but I could not get a good read. I had no idea what he was going to tell us. We gathered around a big table and David pulled out the map of the area he had searched. He pointed to various places on the map where he flew and why he spent so much time circling back in a particular area. He said the water was clear, but that he did not find my Mark.

David had a gentle disposition, and it was a calm conversation. After he explained where and why he searched and was unable to find Mark, I bombarded him with questions. I spilled over with all sorts of questions and scenarios. "What about this? And what about that? How many islands are out there?" And so many other questions. This poor man was so gracious with my questioning and sat politely listening for several minutes.

Then he finally folded his hands, placed them gently on the table, and softly said to me, "Nancy, there's a chance now that we may never find him."

Bang! Once again, my brain felt like a gong hit forcefully with a mallet. *What? Those words could not be said! That can't be possible.* I wanted to slap his face for saying those horrible words. Not in my worst nightmare, or most horrific thoughts, did I think he would *never* be found.

Confusion rushed in. I flung forward toward David stunned and challenging him, my voice lowered, "What? No, no, no. What do you mean *never* find him?" David described things saying this, that, and the other. Ugly things, while being as sensitive as possible, about what the sea might do to a body in the water after five days. He also said there may be a chance that if Mark washed ashore, he may still be alive but that with the number of miles of land and water to search, would an airplane even be able to see him? It was that kind of conversation. And then he went on to say that if Mark were clinging onto something in the ocean that five days would be too long to survive without fresh water. He was very professional, kind, and sympathetic. But those words, *may never be found,* put me into a daze. Instantly my brain shut down. I never considered that as a possibility. And we ended the conversation.

I slowly pushed my chair away, stood up, and staggered back to the bungalow in disbelief. Disoriented. Bewildered. *Never be found?*

I could deal with Mark dying. I could. But my brain could not process him not being found. I did not cry. Numbness consumed me. It was the worst thing to try to grasp. *Tell me he's dead. But don't tell me we'll never know. Because that wasn't an option.*

So, that night at the bungalow I sank into an even deeper level of desperation unlike the other nights, and unlike I had ever experienced before in my life. How many times in this story have I used the word or synonyms of the word numb? How many levels of numb are there?

I laid down and Sami and I texted our usual short, *I love you, we love you, thinking-about-you texts to each other*. After that, I began to pray.

My sister-in-law, Nancy, back home texted me a page from her prayer book and suggested I pray an ancient traditional novena prayer for impossible requests. It is a continual, devotional, and intentional meditative prayer. I unceasingly requested of God that Mark be found even if he wasn't alive. And I prayed the rosary as well. There was nothing more for me to do. And it was the best thing for me to do. Prayerful meditation brought relief and comfort—it took me away to another place within the confines of the bungalow. Though I nodded off for a few minutes here and there throughout the night while praying, I didn't actually sleep. Each time I dozed off I woke up about ten minutes later checking the time on my phone as I waited for the sun to rise.

I battled through prayers trying not to see the evil face of the sea snickering at me. I had long surrendered. All I wanted from that sea was to have the last wave I heard be the one that brought my Mark to shore.

FOURTEEN

Day 9—Fifth Day Of Search, Sunday, March 3rd

The last time I dozed off before dawn on Sunday an amazing thing happened. It was as vivid, clear, and real as anything. *My* Mark was lying beside me on my left side. I felt warm skin on skin right beside me. There he was for what seemed like many magnificent minutes as we basked in our love for each other. And he whispered in my ear, "They know the location." He said it at least three times. We were comfortable together—warm together. We relished deeply in each other's company. Then, suddenly a noise jolted me awake. With eyes wide open I laid motionless realizing what had happened; what was said, and that my body was still warm on my left side. It was *not* my imagination. It was real. He was there. I rolled over to reach for him, but he was gone. *Where did he go?* It was 6:30 am, about an hour before sunrise. I got up and walked to my brother Dave sleeping outside on the cement bench. I stepped toward him, fuzzy minded, still caught in the tender interlude with Mark, and gently tapped him to wake him up.

"Do you hear that?" I whispered. I thought it might have been the volunteers and that maybe Mark had come ashore. I told Dave about the dream. Or was it a vision? No. It was a *visit.* An extraordinarily intimate visit. "Will you please go out there and see what is happening?"

Dave got up and wandered onto the beach for a few minutes. He came back to the bungalow and reported it was just some drunk people walking around. I told him more about my experience with Mark next to me and how warm and beautiful it was, and that he told me they know the location. Dave was very calm and peaceful listening about the encounter. About an hour later, the sun rose.

I hadn't left the bungalow and beach area since Mark disappeared five days earlier, but it was now Sunday and I wanted to go to church. At about 7:30 am Dave, Patti, and I walked to the village into a small Catholic church. I could barely stand so I slumped inside the pew and quietly wept. The priest and parishioners nodded toward me in reverential sympathy likely knowing that I was the woman from the USA looking for her lost husband. Red hair. Freckles. My photo and story had been in the local newspapers.

The Mass was in Spanish. I only understood random words, but the Catholic Mass is the same worldwide, so I fully comprehended the order of the ceremony, and it pacified me as the familiarity of the prayers and offerings washed over my battered soul.

After church we grabbed a cup of coffee at a shop and walked back to the bungalow. I also told Patti about my beautifully extraordinary visit with Mark that morning, and there was something special in the atmosphere as we walked along together.

When we returned to the trailer park, Kirk and Liz were so excited that I finally left the bungalow, and they wanted to keep it going so they pleaded with me to walk back to the village with them for breakfast. I agreed.

Dave and Patti planned to head out for another day of searching for Mark. They didn't let the words from David the pilot, *may never be found,* deter them from continuing to look for him. They believed he was alive somewhere and planned to stay in Mexico for as long as needed until they found him. Kirk had also said he would stay in Mexico as he could do his line of work from there via phone and the internet.

I hadn't yet told Kirk and Liz about my experience with Mark because they were sleeping when Dave, Patti and I left for church, so I told them about it on our walk into town. We went to Choco Banana, the same restaurant we went to on our second day of surfboarding lessons when Mark had ordered a chocolate shake to help with his sea sickness. The food that Kirk and Liz ordered looked delicious, but I still couldn't eat. I sat with them incognito with sunglasses on and sipped my coffee. When we were ready to pay our bill, the waiter told us the meal had been paid for and pointed toward some folks who recognized me from the news. Their sweet act of kindness moved me.

Within ten steps of leaving the restaurant we heard sirens. Loud sirens. I stiffened. I hadn't heard a siren since we'd been in Sayulita. I froze. I knew in my being that it was something about Mark. I just knew it. We turned to look, and down the street came a fire truck. They must have seen me and before the truck had come to a stop, one of the volunteer firemen we'd come to know jumped out and ran toward us yelling, "We found him! We found his body!"

I shook uncontrollably. My body heaved. I tried to catch my breath and for the first time that week, I cried anguishly out loud. I was relieved and grateful. And I felt so guilty for feeling grateful. I was not glad that my Mark was dead. I was relieved they found him. A myriad of emotions enveloped me. *Oh my god they found his body.* It was so sick and so weird and so twisted. I could not feel any pain that Mark had died yet, because I was so relieved and grateful they found him. It was the most guilty, grateful feeling you could have in your life. Such an odd, horrible, peaceful feeling.

This all happened right in town square on a busy Sunday morning. I don't remember what else he said, except that we needed to drive to Puerto Vallarta because Mexico's Pacific Naval Force was bringing him to their base for me to identify his body.

Kirk, Liz, and I got in the emergency vehicle with the fireman because he was going to drive us to the base, and I said, "We can't just go. We have to go back to the bungalow. We have to get my brother and sister-in-law."

We drove to the bungalow, but Dave and Patti were already gone continuing to search for Mark. I took a chance hoping he had his cell phone. He did.

"Dave, they found his body and we need to go to Puerto Vallarta!"

Dave went wild. I don't know how far down the beach they were, but they were out of eyesight. He and Patti ran back to us in the intense heat. Dave had on his usual black jeans, cowboy hat, and cowboy boots, and when he and Patti reached us, Dave was on the verge of passing out. He got into the fire truck and could barely breathe. I was scared for him. I truly thought he was going to have a heart attack. He was in distress. I told the driver we couldn't leave until Dave was okay. It took several minutes for the fireman to help stabilize Dave's breathing. When Dave was finally okay, the five of us and the fireman made our way, with sirens blaring, for the hour-long ride to the Naval Force Base to identify the body. During the entire somber drive down to the base with little conversation, we all wondered, *Is it Mark? Is it not Mark?* I was praying it was him so there could be some sort of closure instead of *never* finding him.

From the moment we arrived at the gate on the base it felt ugly. The fireman told the gate guards why we were there, and the guards looked upon us with disdain and distrust. I didn't bring my passport. Dave had his, and I'm not sure who else had theirs. I didn't even think to bring mine. The guards interrogated us, through the fireman as our interpreter, and eventually they let us on the base. The fireman told us that the body had not yet arrived at the marina—that it was still in transit from where the Navy boat retrieved it. He said 'the body' because even though he initially announced to us that they'd found Mark's body, I still had to positively identify him.

The fireman explained that because of the local media attention and the consulate involvement, more organized searching had begun the last couple of days. Not with search boats, helicopters, or airplanes, but ramped up searching with more local volunteers south of Sayulita. The fireman informed us that two fishermen had found a body about ten miles south of where Mark disappeared, and they contacted the Naval Force. Dave spoke with the fireman separately, and was told that it was a trained spotter with binoculars standing high on the cliffs in the bay in the private area, where he and Patti had previously walked to, but couldn't access, who saw a body in the water several hundred yards out from shore, and that *he* was the one who contacted the Naval Force. It could have been either scenario, with the fishermen finding the body, or a spotter on the cliffs, but it doesn't matter, in the end it was the fishermen who waited next to the body for the Naval Force to arrive and secure the body for identification.

The military police (MPs) at the guard shack had us sit in a grassy area to wait for further instructions. No chairs. Just an open grassy area off to the side of the shack. We wondered how it was all going to play out. Were we going to a morgue? They didn't do anything for us. Just five people from the USA sitting and waiting on the grass. The MPs, holding their big guns, hung around the shack several feet away, patrolling, talking, and gesturing amongst themselves persistently leering our way with suspicion in their eyes—as if we were criminals. The fireman who drove us had gone into a nearby building. After countless minutes he came out and approached us. With a disturbed look in his eyes he said, "The boat has arrived, but they can't take the body off the boat. You have to identify him on the boat."

"What? What are you talking about?" I challenged.

"Since they don't know that it's him, they can't take an unidentified body off the boat due to laws dealing with international waters."

My mind raced. "Um, okay." But I didn't know what that meant. *Was there a suitable place on the boat to do such a thing?* I had no idea what we were in for. The fireman stayed with us as we continued waiting on the grass. Nothing to eat. No water offered to us in the sweltering heat of the day.

We were so confused and decided we needed a plan about calling home if it turns out it was Mark's body. I got on my cell phone and called my sister Joanne saying something like, "We have news. Something is happening." I didn't offer any more information, but I told her I wanted Jacob, Lucas, Sami, and our mom to be together at the house for any new information. It was much more complicated than that, but that's all I remember.

The day before, as I agonized inside the bungalow struggling between the fine line of hoping against hope that David the pilot would find Mark, and trying to quell the simultaneous surges of despair that flooded my mind, I called my friend, Susan, who worked with a family therapist. I asked her to please call her therapist and ask how, if Mark is found dead, do I tell my children? I did not want to damage them for life. I just wanted to make sure that if it were Mark's body that I would tell them the best way with the least amount of damage. The thought of making that call to my children repulsed me to my core. The therapist told Susan to tell me that I should tell them straight out. Just like ripping off a band-aid. Just say it, just say your dad died, they found his body.

Finally, a few MPs brandishing their rifles approached us and one of them told the fireman we needed to follow them. The MPs flanked the five of us on all sides as they led us to the boat. What an eerie feeling. We zigzagged across the base to the dock area. When we stopped at the water's edge, one of the MPs pointed out to the water at the boat anchored to the far end of the long T-shaped dock. It was a smaller boat, not a ship, used obviously for such things as search-and-recovery missions and who knows what else.

The MPs continued marshalling us as we marched down the long wooden T-shaped dock, about the length of half a city block. When we came to the T the MP in charge stopped, gestured toward me, and said to the fireman that only I could continue to the end of the dock where the boat was anchored, as it had to be a family member to identify the body. I shrunk back. *Bang the gong again against my brain.* The five of us looked at one another stunned, and the others in an effort to protect me, argued against me being the one to identify the body. I vacillated as to whether or not I wanted to be the one as well. Not that I was afraid to view a dead body, but my mind went back to what David the pilot said about what happens to a body after it has been in the ocean for five days. It was fear of the unknown. *How would I ever be able to get whatever I was going to see out of my mind?* I was afraid of what I was going to see. I didn't know how to prepare myself. Dave understood the fear in my eyes and immediately told the fireman that he was my brother and that he would do it—that he wanted to go with me. The fireman explained that to the MPs and they gave the okay since he was my brother.

At least three MPs, the fireman, Dave, and I walked slowly down the dock— my hollow stare transfixed on the boat. My legs felt heavy and robotic. I noticed a monster-sized black plastic bag at the rear of the boat. We reached the farthest end of the dock and noticed the air itself had suddenly changed. It became unholy. A couple of the MPs grabbed both of my arms. It felt like I was under arrest, but I believe they were there to hold me up in case I fainted.

The MP told the fireman that when they open the bag, they would motion for Dave to come aboard to identify the body. We were about two steps away from the boat. Close enough to observe what was happening.

Three sailors on the boat walked to the giant black bag and one of them bent down to unzip it. He fumbled around for a minute or so and then spoke in Spanish to the other two men shaking his head, and he moved away and stood off to the side. A second sailor approached the bag, stooped over it and was obviously struggling with something on the bag for a couple more minutes. He too stood up and walked away, then motioned to the fireman to come over to inform him what was happening.

The fireman came back to us and said, "They can't get the zipper open."

"Oh my god, are you kidding me?" I put my head in my hands. *Are you kidding me!*

Dave and I looked back at Patti, Kirk, and Liz left behind on the other part of the dock shaking our heads in disgust. A third sailor tried to unzip the bag, and then others. It went on for about ten grueling minutes. I thought, *Just cut the damn thing open!*

"Can't you just cut it open?" I pleaded.

They said they couldn't cut it open in case the body wasn't Mark's, and that it would then be considered unlawful in some way.

When they finally got the zipper open, they saw that the body was upside down. At that point I turned away. The MPs still holding my arms.

Somehow, after about another ten minutes they turned the body around. I don't know how they did it and I didn't want to know.

Dave went aboard the boat. He looked inside the bag for the longest time, and then turned to me with intense pain in his eyes and said, "I don't know if it's him."

What! Our eyes locked tightly on each other. I felt so sad that he had to be the one to look inside the bag. Now I was angry. Not at Dave. Not at him at all. But at this dreadful situation. Waiting. Waiting. Waiting. My poor brother was exposed to something evidently upsetting and he couldn't even tell me if it was Mark or not. I could not believe this nightmare that wouldn't end with everything from the day of Mark's disappearance to now all being handled so disrespectfully. In the United States, we would have been treated with care and concern and brought to a sanitized morgue to try to identify my husband. But this! This dock. This boat. The bag in the thick heat of the day. It was unsacred. At that point I couldn't take it anymore. I needed to know. I couldn't fathom what I was about to see. So often it is the difficult things we see that tend to stay in the forefront of our mind even more so than the beautiful things. And I did not want my memory of Mark tainted like that. I did not want what I was about to see to be the main thing I would think of—forever and always. I was so afraid of that.

But I had enough. I pushed the MPs away from me. They tried to stop me, but I got onto the boat, looked down into the bag and then understood Dave's anguish and inability to make a positive identification. I looked at two or three different things. Then, I saw the infamous railroad scar extending from his inside thigh down to his calf due to a softball injury from many years ago. I confirmed with the captain of the boat that it was *my* Mark. They asked if I was certain. I said yes.

The MPs then escorted us back to Patti, Kirk, and Liz. As Dave and I walked, we encouraged each other saying, "That was just flesh. It wasn't Mark. He's in our hearts. He's in heaven."

We reached the others. We hugged. We cried. I said, "We *have to* pray together right now." And we prayed the Our Father right there on the dock.

One of the MPs instructed the fireman to drive us a few miles away to the State Attorney's Office in Puerto Vallarta. Why there? We weren't told.

We got to the building and three armed guards approached us, and in Spanish one of them told the fireman that I needed to follow them inside.

"Somebody's coming with me, aren't they?" I asked.

The fireman asked the guard.

The guard responded, "No." That only the fireman could be with me as my interpreter.

I bristled. I looked at Dave, Patti, Kirk, and Liz. They stood outside watching as yet another set of heavily armed guards walked me and the fireman out of sight and into the building, while a few other armed guards stood watch outside in the oppressive heat over the four of them.

During that time, Dave called home to our local funeral home director, Dan Delmore, of Gearty-Delmore Funeral Chapels in Robbinsdale, to find out if he knew of a reputable funeral home in Puerto Vallarta. Dan was aware of Mark's disappearance with all the news stories back home, and he gave Dave instructions as to how to move ahead with a funeral home nearby.

The guards brought the fireman and me into a small, stark, windowless, white-washed sterile room and left us there closing the door behind them. There were three metal desks with workers at each one, a TV mounted high in a corner, and a telephone on the wall. There wasn't a chair for me or the fireman to sit on. We stood before a middle-aged Spanish speaking woman at one of the desks. Her computer faced the TV and there was a soccer game playing. I stood before her; my hands folded together to hide their trembling as she asked the fireman interrogating questions for me to answer.

The reason we needed to go to the highly secured building is that since I was able to identify Mark in international waters, the Mexican government needed detailed information as to the events occurring on the day he disappeared.

The authorities had also moved Mark's body to the office building, and he was in a room next to ours.

As the interrogation moved along, the woman split her time asking me questions with the help of the fireman interpreting, while typing and looking up at the TV to keep an eye on the soccer game. Multiple times during those arduous proceedings she turned to the fireman, motioned toward the next room, and making an awful face said, "Necesitas mover el cuerpo!" (You need to move the body!). "Huele mal!" (He smells bad!). "Apesta." (He stinks!). "Esta es una oficina. No temenos refrigeracíon. Necesitas mover el cuerpo!" (This is an office. We don't have refrigeration. You need to move the body!).

The first time the fireman told me what she said I nearly vomited on her desk in disgust with what she was saying. She made those comments at least three more times. Yes, she was correct about the unpleasant smell, but she was talking about my husband! And *her* government is the one who brought us there. What was I supposed to do? I couldn't help that it was a

Sunday, and the woman was angry because my husband's death interfered with her precious soccer game. I felt like an annoyance. My legs trembled as I continued standing before her in that dreary room. I finally rested my hand on the desk so that I didn't fall to my knees.

I asked the fireman to ask her if she knew she was referring to my dead husband. He did. But she didn't care. There was no kindness, concern, or compassion whatsoever. She was so flippant. As if I'd lost my dog. But even then, that would have been a tragedy certainly calling for compassion. She was more interested in the soccer game. I asked for a chair and after about fifteen minutes someone brought in a cold metal one for me.

The woman continued drilling me, with the help of the fireman, repeatedly asking and re-asking ludicrous questions about why we were in Sayulita, where I was when Mark went into the water, his disappearance, and the hours afterward as we searched for him until nightfall. It was so emotionally taxing. It seemed like I was *on trial.* Then the fireman received an emergency call and told me he had to leave.

"What!" That was my breakdown. I just started bawling. I grabbed his arm, "You can't leave. She is yelling at me because my husband's body smells! Where is someone from the consulate? Who is going to help me?"

The fireman radioed back saying he couldn't leave me yet, and he ended up staying. He then called our consulate contact from the phone on the wall in the room and handed me the receiver. I was beside myself explaining the rudeness and apathy of the woman, offensive cross-questioning, no chair for me to sit on until I finally asked for one, and over and over again telling me that my husband's body stinks and that they need to move the body. The appalling ordeal lasted about an hour and a half.

The consulate representative moved quickly to have Mark's body brought to a local funeral home. The armed guards then walked me and the fireman outside. I told Dave, Patti, Kirk, and Liz what happened inside, and the fireman said he really needed to get back to Sayulita, and he left. We were left standing there with no transportation to the funeral home. We had the address written down and stood looking at one another perplexed. Patti, in her mild-mannered way, then walked up to one of the gun-carrying guards, showed him the address to the funeral home, and he called a taxi for us.

As we waited for the taxi, I looked at the others and stared right through them. I walked away and thought, *I have to call my children outside this horrible, horrible place.* I knew now was the time to call home and tell my children their dad had drowned. I figured by now my mom and children were at the house waiting for my phone call, as a result of my earlier call to Joanne, while we waited on the grass at the Naval Base. There was no other time to call them, not only because I was reeling in the trauma surrounding the identification of Mark's body, but everything had moved so quickly, like a whirlwind, from the excruciatingly painful fiasco at the base, to when we were transported a short distance away to the state office building where I stood trapped in the disgusting, insensitive interrogation room. With my insides crumbling, I called my mom. My voice quivered and throat tightened. I was her broken daughter who needed my mom. Though she struggled with Alzheimer's she was very much aware of our dire situation. She told me that word had spread like wildfire with the earlier news of a development, and the house quickly filled again to standing room only with people waiting outside. I asked her to please go into Mark's and my bedroom with Jacob, Lucas, and Sami, and to close the door and put the phone on speaker. She did and I told Jacob, Lucas, and Sami that their dad died—that they found his body. I ripped off the band-aid just like the therapist suggested. There was silence, there was sobbing, and there was much exasperation on both ends of the phone.

When the taxi arrived, it was one meant for four people at best including the driver. We all looked at each other shaking our heads saying, "Really?" The guard could have told them how many people would be riding. That was just one more turn of the knife in already open wounds for all of us. The five of us piled in and sat scrunched and unable to move during the several mile ride. On the way to the funeral home, I told the others we needed to find out about flying Mark home for a casket burial. Would we buy a casket in Mexico? How would they fly him home? With us? Another day?

We arrived at the funeral home and the director greeted us. Kirk was able to speak broken Spanish and English with him—Spanglish—enough to understand that Mark's body had arrived. After a short while, the director handed me papers to complete. When he saw that I wrote down Mark's date of death as the date he disappeared on February 26, 2013, he said no, that the date of death is the date they found his body.

We argued back and forth with Kirk translating in Spanglish.

"No, no, no!" I said. "He didn't die today."

"It doesn't matter," the director insisted, "the date has to be today, March 3, 2013."

Again, another bang of the gong against my brain. *Are you kidding me?* But I was desensitized by then. Weak. Beaten down. Empty. I did not have any more fight in me. I just wanted to be gone from that place and back home with our children. So, I reluctantly continued completing the paperwork and resentfully wrote down March 3rd. while Kirk conversed with the director a few feet away. A couple of minutes later Kirk walked slowly toward me frowning.

"What's wrong?" I asked.

"They have to cremate him."

"No, no, no." I said. "That is not our plan. We're going to transport the body and we're going to bury him."

"The director told me no." Kirk said.

"Yes, we are!" I demanded.

Kirk sorrowfully explained, "No, it's the law. Because of the condition of the body, he must be cremated."

Dave connected again with Dan Delmore, the funeral director back home, and Dan confirmed that the funeral home in Puerto Vallarta was reputable, and that the director was correct in saying they must cremate Mark's body before flying him back home.

Dave was an angel. I appreciated so much that he was getting things organized back home and that he was doing so with a kind man whom we respected. I found that home connection so comforting amid our despicable nightmare.

Yes, Dave was an angel and so were Patti, Kirk, and Liz during those horrid days—all in their own special ways.

Because Kirk spoke Spanglish, he and I then followed the funeral director upstairs to choose a box for the ashes with the cremation payment due right then. I looked at all of the boxes in disbelief and completely distraught that my Mark had to be cremated, and just wanted to buy the cheapest one they had knowing I'd buy a more suitable one when I returned home. I didn't want to give them any more money than I needed to.

I didn't have a credit card or cash on me at the time, and Kirk graciously said, "Don't worry about it, Nancy. I'll take care of it."

I was so grateful for him. What a loving act of kindness. In a few short minutes we learned that Mark couldn't be buried, he had to be cremated, and now, 'give us the money.'

The director said they would do a required autopsy before the cremation. The outcome of the autopsy would provide critical information for insurance purposes. Did Mark have a heart attack? Was it accidental? The director informed us he could do the cremation that evening, as they do 24-hour cremations, and we could pick up Mark's ashes on Monday. On the one hand I was relieved they could do it so quickly, but on the other hand, it sounded so callous.

I told Dave to tell Dan Delmore I'd be flying home on Tuesday with Mark's ashes, and wanted the wake that same week on Thursday with a Friday morning funeral. Dan told Dave that there was no chance we were going to get the ashes out of the country that quickly in time for a Friday funeral.

Dave told Dan, "Well, Nancy said it's going to happen so let's just go with it." And Dan told Dave if anyone were going to get it done, it would be Nancy.

I believe the reason it worked so quickly is that we were already dealing with the consulate, and Dave and Patti had gone into town to fax them our documents earlier in the week, so the final paperwork was easier to process. Had Mark drowned and been found on the same day, more than likely the paperwork wouldn't have processed so quickly.

Before we caught a shuttle back to Sayulita, we stopped at a restaurant and that was the first time I had nibbled on anything more than crackers for five days. I nibbled on chips instead. Our plan was to go back to the bungalow for another day to pack up our things, and leave for home the following day on Tuesday. On the way to the airport, we planned to pick up Mark's ashes, death certificate, and other papers needed for flying him home.

Dave shared how disappointed he was that he and Patti were not the people to have spotted him, because they were near that same private area where the resort gate guard wouldn't allow them access. Though they likely wouldn't have seen him on the other days, just knowing he and Patti had searched near where Mark was ultimately found, made him wish they would've been the one's to see him first. Dave said how fortunate it was that the current brought Mark around to the next bay, otherwise he would have been swept straight out to sea and perhaps never found.

We were mostly silent on the shuttle ride back to Sayulita. At one point Liz looked at me and started crying. "I just can't believe it. I can't believe he died. I can't believe God would do that to you after you saved that man's life the same day that Mark drowned."

I looked at her baffled, "What are you talking about?" I had totally forgotten about the incident with the surfer face down on the beach that day.

We talked more about that morning and how great it was that she saw the man first, but no one else did. We revisited how I helped him, and then the doctor stitched him up. We surmised that he probably went back to Nuevo Vallarta unaware of what happened to Mark later that day, and that there was no opportunity for me to save my own husband—*my* Mark.

It ended up being five days of moments upon moments from hell. One thing after another kept happening, and I would think, *This just can't be real. It couldn't possibly be real.* I truly wanted someone to sock me in the head and wake me up. This is stuff you read about. It couldn't be real—I found myself playing a part in a disturbing nightmare. That is how I felt. It was so surreal.

The next CaringBridge post words were mine that I texted to Kim saying we found Mark today, but not in the way in which we had prayed. I said we received the miracle we were hoping for in finding him, but not the outcome we had prayed for that he would be alive. We are working to bring Mark's body home to our family, and appreciate all the love, support, and prayers as they have helped more than you know. And I ended the post with love, from the Stoneberg family.

The TV news and newspapers back home reported that Mark's body was found after nearly a week-long search.

One source quoted me saying, "It is with a heavy heart that we inform you that the body of Mark Stoneberg was located this morning off the coast of Mexico."

A local news station reported that people took to Twitter to express their sadness, that the entire city of Robbinsdale grieved for our family, and that I asked for privacy during this difficult time.

Sami's texts that night had a sound of pained peacefulness. Similar to my feelings when the fireman told me they found Mark's body. Just grateful he was recovered. "We love you mom. See you in a couple of days."

Another night. The sixth in a row of listening to the coldblooded pulse of the sea relentlessly crashing—the ravenous waters that swallowed *our* Mark whole. But now that Mark's body was found, the waves no longer taunted and threatened me. I no longer had to wonder if the last wave I heard was the one that would have brought him ashore. The monotonous jarring left me completely sapped. But I still couldn't sleep and again tossed and turned all night. I couldn't wait to get back home. I ached desperately to be with our children, and wished I were supernatural so I could simply snap my fingers and be instantly back home with them.

FIFTEEN

Day 10—The Day Before Flying Home, Monday, March 4th

Early that morning, I called Jacob to give him the flight information. He said, "Mom, nobody else can pick you up from the airport. Mom, please, please, don't let anyone else come with us. It has to be me, Lucas, and Sami."

I told him of course and that I wanted to be only with them as well.

David the pilot returned to Sayulita on Monday morning to offer his condolences, and told us that he had been searching the previous day in the same area where Mark had been found. I asked him why he thought Mark finally surfaced after five days. We had previously discussed Mark's height, weight, and muscle mass and he believed likely the reason was because he was 6'5", weighed 220 pounds with very little body fat, and that body fat creates buoyancy. Since muscle is twice as heavy as fat, he remained under water longer. When I told David that Mark had titanium in his body from knee surgery, he confirmed that would also have restricted his surfacing, and said it was nothing less than a miracle that he was found.

Later that day, Dave, Patti, Kirk, Liz, and I each wrote a note to Mark and placed them in one bottle and corked it tight. The tide was still rough. Dave walked a fair distance into the water and threw it. The white water washed it quickly back in. He walked out further and threw it again, only to have the waves push it back again as if the ocean spat at us not allowing us to have peace. It was bizarre that Dave could not get it out far enough— over and over again relentlessly throwing it further out. Just when he got it past the break another set of waves rose up and washed it back in. It seemed like the ocean was toying with us. The only words for any of us to each other were an emphatic, "Are you kidding me!"

All we wanted was to have closure. We couldn't even get a bottle out into the water with our words of love to Mark in the sea that took his last breath. It wouldn't let us. Once again, we just wanted to have peace, and this beast would not let us. It was so sad, frustrating, and heart crushing. It seemed like the sea was mocking us and relishing in the travesty as if taking another gratifying morsel of our very being.

Dave finally ran about a half-mile to the northside of the beach, climbed out onto the boulders and threw the bottle from there. He said he believed he threw it out far enough and that it made it beyond any waves that would wash it back in. We all walked back to the bungalow together emotionally and physically wasted.

A little while later, I walked with Liz and Kirk to the boulders on the north side as they wanted to build a cairn—a small, stacked, stone memorial for my Mark in the sacred area where he disappeared. I was entirely spent and didn't have the energy to join in, so I just sat on the beach and solemnly watched them reverently pile little flat rocks they found on the beach—balancing them just right to create a uniquely beautiful tiny stone stairway pointing to heaven.

We walked back to the bungalow and then the five of us, Kirk, Liz, David, Patti, and I strode joylessly to the village one last time before leaving the next day. The others needed to eat. My appetite had not yet returned, but I managed to snack again on some chips.

The afternoon passed by as I sat inside the bungalow staring emptily at the wall. I just wanted to be home with my children.

Around 4:30 pm Patti came to me and said the locals had planned a beachside celebration of life, and farewell for us, near the location where Mark went into the water. I was surprised.

"Really?" I muttered.

"Yes, and they're gathering right now."

I started to walk out of the bungalow, but Patti stopped me saying, "Nancy, I think you might want to change into something else."

"Why?" I looked down at myself. I had on jeans, a t-shirt, and sandals.

Patti said, "There's a lot of people out there and I think it would be more appropriate if you put on a dress if you saw what was happening."

I peeked out the door at the beach. I was humbled beyond measure watching the parade of people coming from all directions onto the beach. People wore their best beachwear carrying bouquets of flowers likely picked from the local forest, and musicians brought their instruments. "You're right. I'll put on a sun dress."

I put on the blue and green floral dress that Mark liked the best on me. He liked how it accentuated my blue eyes and red hair.

The five of us walked across the sand with one another to the ceremony. As we strolled toward the group, the sound of a conch shell horn announced prayers into the atmosphere as that is their tradition for a beach memorial ceremony.

There had to have been a hundred or more people. The entire beach was filled with people we knew from the previous days search-and-rescue efforts, but mostly with folks we'd never seen before.

They placed me on a chair facing the ocean and across from a bamboo table covered with flowers. Patti and Liz sat on each side of me. I settled in the chair gathering my thoughts trying to wrap my head around what was happening. Out of nowhere a dog came and sat right beside me.

Kirk stood a few feet away from me flagging me down to get my attention. He had a look of astonishment on his face—his wide eyes and forward gaze looking alternately at me and then down at the dog.

I looked at the dog and back at Kirk puzzled. *What?*

He quickly came over to me and pointed at the dog, whispering, "That's the dog!"

"What?"

"That's the dog! The G-O-D dog."

Chills rushed through my body. *No way.* I looked down at the dog again sitting calmly next to me, then back at Kirk. He nodded his head yes. I stared vacantly back at him not knowing what to do with that information. My attention was then quickly drawn to the sound of musicians joining together. The air filled with traditional Mexican instruments—drums, flutes, maracas, and guitars that started precisely at 5:15 pm—the time when *our* Mark had disappeared five days earlier.

A local pastor officiated the service offering prayers for Mark, me, and all our loved ones and friends. He didn't know Mark, but he knew the dire circumstances of the preceding several days and spoke tender and loving words.

After his sermon, the music played on and people sang while a procession of people approached me holding white tea light candles in glass holders offering their condolences, and placed the candles on the bamboo table. Some stood, some bent over, and some were on their knees so they could be eye level with me. One woman put a fresh leigh of flowers around my neck. Another woman presented me with a beautifully colored hand tooled bronze cross that she made specifically for me. The ceremony continued until sunset to commemorate when the search ended that first agonizing night. I don't know when the dog left, but I never saw it again.

We all went to bed early that night. It was the final night of Sami's texting before I flew out the next day. "We love you mom. Can't wait to see you."

I yearned deeply to be with her, Jacob, and Lucas. To hug them and cry with them. To just *be* with them.

I was so shattered and torn and thought for certain I'd finally be able to sleep until sunrise. But no, the monotonous lashing of the waves kept me awake like the force of a bludgeon, which in fact is what the wave that hit Mark turned out to be. He was gone in a blink of an eye. Stolen by a ghostly spineless thief. Captured before our very eyes.

SIXTEEN

Day 11—Returning Home, Tuesday March 5th

It was mid-morning. I packed my bag to go home haphazardly piling up unfolded clothes. Neatness and order did not matter. Neatness and order had been stripped from my being. I stared quizzically at Mark's clothes. *Do I need to pack them? He's not going to wear them anymore. Yes, I must bring them home. Especially his shorts that I laid with and used as my 'pillow' each night.*

Unlike my clothes that I tossed into my suitcase, I meticulously folded Mark's clothing holding up each item and breathing in his scent. I found his cell phone in his duffel bag, which was odd, because we'd looked for it previously but couldn't find it. I called his phone repeatedly just so I could listen to his voice recording. I replayed one of his messages on my phone over and over again that he left for me when I was creating the playlist when he said, "I was just thinking. Get that Carrie Underwood song I like. You know the one I'm talking about…when she beats up the car. Talk to you later. Love ya. Bye." The song is called "Before He Cheats," and I could tell he was eating an apple when he left the message because I know what he sounds like when he is chewing one. He had a certain unique way of eating an apple, and most of the time it was an endearing sound; however, when I wasn't happy with him, it annoyed me. I would give anything for that annoyance now.

When I picked up one of Mark's XXL V-neck undershirts, I thought back to the other one of his that I'd worn and became blood-stained when I helped save the elderly surfer's life the morning of Mark's disappearance. I thought about Liz's remark as to why God allowed Mark to die that very same day. I wondered the same thing.

I shuffled over to his sock-stuffed shoes that I had intentionally left untouched from when he removed them right before going body surfing one last time before dinner. I wanted them right where he set them so he could return and put them back on. It was haunting to look at them every day and night, but it was necessary. If someone would have tried to move them, I would have screamed, "You can't touch them! They have to stay there. They're waiting for Mark!" I then removed the socks, reached in, and found his wallet in one shoe, but nothing in the other. I then embraced his shoes before placing them gently in his duffel bag, and then zipped it up.

Soon afterward, the five of us rode down to Puerto Vallarta in a large black SUV driven by a local taxi driver. We told the driver we first needed to go to the consulate in Nuevo Vallarta to pick up the death and cremation certificates in order to transport Mark's ashes on the airplane, and then to the funeral home in Puerto Vallarta to pick up his ashes. The driver offered his condolences and told us about a brother or best friend, I don't remember which one, who had drowned in those same waters. He had been a surfer born and raised in Sayulita.

In Nuevo Vallarta, the consulate representative that had been assisting us the previous several days, presented me with the documents. I read the death certificate and the results of the autopsy revealed that Mark had drowned. And I believe he drowned immediately from the impact of the first big wave because he never surfaced.

When we reached the funeral home in Puerto Vallarta, the same funeral director from two days before greeted us and presented me with the plain wooden box holding Mark's ashes. I looked at him emotionless remembering his last words from that day, "We're open 24-hours and can cremate him anytime." The five of us remained speechless as we walked out the door.

We had some time before we needed to be at the airport, so we asked the taxi driver to drop all of us off at Dave and Patti's hotel near the airport in Puerto Vallarta. They had to stay another night because all the flights were booked that day. We had a couple of beers together at the hotel and set the box with Mark's ashes next to us. We placed an extra beer for Mark beside the box and offered toasts to him.

When it came time for Kirk, Liz, and me to take another taxi to the airport, I began to place the box with Mark's ashes inside my carry-on suitcase, the suitcase that Mark thought was so cool because it fit under the seat, and I emotionally lost it. Tears gushed. My stomach churned, and my crushed heart felt like it was ready to burst into pieces. *What an unthinkable thing this is. Mark, I am so sorry.* The five of us hugged one another tight. I gathered myself and shuffled to the taxi—my feet feeling like they were made of lead. Our flight was at 3:45 pm and by 8:30 pm I'd be embracing my children at the Minneapolis airport.

Earlier in the day, one of my very dear friends had called Patti to tell her how to prepare me for leaving my 'safe place' where I had been sheltered near the village and the bungalow area—the only small area I'd been in for days embraced by people who loved me, and others in the area who knew of my situation. My friend had been a flight attendant for many years, and she wanted me to be aware of the emotional insanity that was going to occur with me walking inside the airport and leaving without Mark alive. She wanted me to know the anxiety of being thrown out into the general population where no one knew I carried my husband's ashes in my carry-on, and that I wouldn't be treated any differently than anyone else at the airport. She wanted me prepared for going through security with the thorough checking of the documents, the box which held Mark's ashes, and extensive questions by the security staff.

When Patti told me what she had said, I held on to every word. I was grateful for my friend's support as none of that even crossed my mind. And she was right. Being informed proved vital. I tried to prepare myself mentally, but nothing could have prepared me for the dizziness I experienced stepping into the airport without Mark by my side. I went into sensory overload with the commotion and buzzing of travelers moving every which way under the bright harshly lit ceiling lights that reflected on the white-on-white shiny walls; that ricocheted off the metal columns and glossy tile floor. It felt like an assault from another dimension—a clash of societies—after having spent several days in the quiet, humble, village surroundings and burrowed in the bungalow. I took a step back and stopped to get my bearings and wits about me. I'd been inside that airport numerous times before, yet I didn't fully comprehend the complicated depths of feelings I'd have with suddenly needing to deal with everything that would happen 'out there,' and not feel safe anymore; and that the myriads of people inside that cold sterile environment were oblivious to my family's tragedy. Kirk and Liz must have felt the same emotions, but they didn't say anything to me. Thankfully, we were with one another every step of the way.

The baggage check-in moved swiftly but the line to pass through security was slow and long. When my turn came to check in, my hands trembled as I presented my ticket and passport to the security agent, and he approved my documents. When I handed him Mark's passport and the death and cremation certificates showing I came there with him, and was now leaving with him in a box, my whole body shook. The agent's unsympathetic questioning nauseated me. *Really, again?* I understood he had a job to do but it felt so unkind. I eventually made it past security and then…the final blow. I placed the box with *my* Mark's ashes on the belt to be scanned by the x-ray machine—as if it were just another everyday item to scrutinize for potential danger.

Kirk, Liz, and I waited in the airport terminal for our flight to be called. I sat curled into a ball on a chair shrouded in the Mexican blanket staring vacantly at the floor with Mark's ashes nestled next to me in my carry-on bag. The sounds around me suddenly changed. I looked up and noticed a Delta pilot walking toward me looking straight into my eyes. He walked very slowly yet precisely. I stared vacantly back at him. He reached me and dropped down to one knee with obvious sorrow in his eyes. He placed his hand upon my knee and slowly removed his cap saying, "Mrs. Stoneberg, I'm so very sorry for your loss. I'm a member of your parish back home and I heard about what happened to your husband. Everyone is praying for you and your family. I'm here to bring you and Mark home safely to your family."

Tears spilled down my face. My heart overwhelmed by his kindness; his gentleness. There before me knelt a man of distinction from my own church of all places, honoring Mark, me, and our children. All I could say was, "Thank you." No other words could be found. I have no idea how he knew I was going to be on the flight.

We boarded the airplane, and when I finished buckling myself into my coach seat next to Liz sitting with my head down, I heard a woman saying,

"Ma'am, ma'am." I looked up and there were three flight attendants looking at me.

One of them said, "Ma'am, could you come with us?"

I was completely stunned and suddenly anxious. "Why?"

"Could you please just come with us?"

I looked at all of them puzzled and had a terrible feeling like I was doing something wrong. Thinking maybe I wasn't supposed to have Mark in my carry-on with me. It seemed highly official with three flight attendants standing over me. "Ma'am, the captain explained to us what has happened to you and your husband; we would like you to come with us. We would like to bring you up to first class so we can take care of you."

I was overcome by their care and concern. I accepted the offer, and they escorted me up to first class and placed me by the window next to a woman sitting in the aisle seat. I was thankful I had the window seat. I put my bag with Mark's ashes under the seat in front of me, pulled the Mexican blanket over me, and rested my head against the cabin wall staring blankly out the window thinking only of my children and what that reunion was going to be like.

I thought, *How am I going to go home and be there without their dad? How am I going to look at them?* The aching pain was unbearable. I just wanted to go to sleep and wake up realizing it was all just a bad, bad dream.

After a brief time, the woman asked me why they escorted me up to first class, and I said, "I arrived here with my husband and now I'm leaving with him in my suitcase." And I told her the story.

She looked at me spellbound asking, "How could all that be possible?"

I just looked at her as I lowered and shook my head pondering the same thing. I again leaned my head against the window and tried my best to fall asleep and wish it all away. All I kept thinking about was my children. I needed to be with them. I wanted to be with them so badly, yet I was afraid to be with them. It was a hideous two-edged sword. I didn't know if I could bear it. I was so afraid of how much more badly it was going to hurt with the melding of our collective anguish. I sat straight up, my head spun, and my chest and throat tightened. I began to hyperventilate and felt like I was going to pass out. I eventually steadied myself and tried again to relax. I experienced a few more bouts of anxiety on the four-hour flight as I thought about needing to be home, but terrified at the same time.

We arrived in Minneapolis and Kirk, Liz, and I retrieved our bags at the baggage claim. When I'd spoken to Jacob two days prior about picking us up, I asked him to wait for us in the SUV at the terminal as I didn't want to experience our sorrowful reunion inside the airport.

The three of us walked outside and I immediately spotted Mark's black SUV at the curb. My heart raced. Jacob, Lucas, and Sami got out and we hugged tightly. The four of us moved to the back seat while Kirk and Liz drove us. My children and I held one another and wept as we rode to Kirk's house to drop off him and Liz, and then Jacob drove us home from there. Our family and friends who had been there for so many days, had left us alone to grieve in private.

I put Mark's ashes in our bedroom and next to it placed the handmade bronze cross the woman in Mexico made for me, and set my things in the porch bedroom. I could not fathom sleeping in our bedroom without Mark by my side. That was the only bedroom we had shared together, and that bed stayed in the exact same spot throughout our marriage. It was so painful to even go in there much less think about sleeping in there.

I went to the kitchen for a glass of water. Jacob, Lucas, and Sami stood lined up next to each other against the counter. They moved slowly away from one another with saddened eyes to reveal a burnt hole in the countertop that was not there before our vacation.

It turned out that while Kirk, Liz, Mark, and I were partying in the village on our first night in Sayulita just eleven days prior, our children at home had hosted a party of their own in our house with about thirty or so people. Someone brought a hookah pipe, and somehow it fell over off its stand and a coal from the pipe melted a square inch hole in the middle of our laminate kitchen countertop.

They told me how fearful and worried sick they were of Mark and me when we returned home as there was no fixing it. The hole was in the middle of our counter and they would have had to cut it out. They googled how to repair melted laminate but there was no solution. I shrugged it off as something trivial considering Mark's death. And the three of them agreed that after my phone call on Tuesday night, no one cared about the countertop anymore.

The four of us; Jacob, Lucas, Sami, and I snuggled and slept together all night on the same big inflatable bed in the porch bedroom. My mom had lived with us for years, and the porch bedroom was hers, but she had recently moved out and had taken her bed with her.

SEVENTEEN

First Full Day At Home, Wednesday, March 6th

The CaringBridge post, which was the final one on our page, informed people of the visitation on Thursday, March 7, 2013, at the Gearty-Delmore Robbinsdale Chapel, with the Mass of Christian Burial at Sacred Heart Church at 10 am on Friday March 8, 2013.

I got up early the next morning in a stupor and shuffled into the kitchen. I felt the need to create something familiar. I had a longing for normalcy. I opened the refrigerator and grabbed a huge stack of uncooked bacon that I noticed the night before that Kim's husband, Joe, had provided for us. It was about ten pounds of bacon from a bulk supplier, and I proceeded to cook it. All of it. I wanted the smell of bacon because to me the smell of bacon meant family, it meant hominess and warmth, and it was a smell we all loved. I wanted my children to smell something good. I figured people would be coming and going all day, and knew that if the plate was sitting on the counter that every bit of it would get eaten.

After all the bacon was cooked, I crawled back onto the inflatable mattress with my children. They eventually got up and went to other parts of the house, but I ended up staying in bed most of the day. When family and friends came over, they had to visit with me in the porch bedroom where I laid physically and mentally immobile.

In the early evening, after friends and family had left, I ventured out of the bedroom and into our dimly lit living room for a change of scenery. That was when I sat curled up next to the fireplace and the song "Mad World" randomly played on my playlist, and when Lucas came running; imploring me to *Turn It Off!* As that was the song he heard in the background on that fateful night of Mark's disappearance when I called home.

EIGHTEEN

Funeral Home Visitation, Thursday, March 7th

I woke up feeling slightly more rested than on any other morning since the tragedy, but still with much broken sleep, and I moved slowly. It was all I could do to try to be strong for my children as I struggled through the basic tasks of showering and getting dressed for the funeral home visitation. I still hadn't eaten much since Mark's disappearance, and Jacob, Lucas, Sami, and I putzed around the house gearing up for the wake at 4 pm.

Mark's sister's, Missy and Donna, were at the house as well and they both apprehensively took on the difficult task of going to the funeral home to meet with Dan Delmore before the wake to get things in order. I am grateful to them for that as they knew I was mentally exhausted and incapable of organizing those details. Donna had driven home to get some things before meeting Missy there, and Missy said she would walk as she needed fresh air. She trudged through the slushy, thawing winter snow trying to avoid icy patches along the one-mile trek. The cloudy overcast weather matched the mood of the day. Missy was further disheartened that her youngest of two sons, Alex, couldn't be at his uncle Mark's funeral. He was in the military and had recently been deployed to South Korea and tried desperately to come home, but was unable get leave. Missy told me later her mind was so jumbled that day that she had struggled to tell Dan Delmore of Mark's middle name. She knew it was an odd spelling of Lawrence and finally remembered it was spelled Lourence.

Donna returned to the funeral home later with two lovely large photo collages that she and her daughter, Melissa, had created to honor Mark. She said it was a blessing to do it as it was the only thing in their lives that they could control regarding Mark's *life*.

When it came time to drive to the funeral home my children and I drove Mark's SUV. We encouraged one another saying, "We can do this." We had a tight bond—a special connection knowing Mark would expect us to hold it together and do it right. A CD rested in the player just as Mark had left it. Metallica's song "One" played on. We cranked up the volume in honor of Mark during the heartbreaking mile drive to the visitation.

I can't remember anything
Can't tell if this is true or dream
Deep down inside I feel to scream
This terrible silence stops me.

From the beginning of the four-hour wake to its ending, the chapel remained filled to overflowing with a continual line outside the door. What an amazing outpouring of love for our family. Dan Delmore said it was one of the largest wakes he had ever seen at their chapel.

The last half hour of the visitation ended with a prayer service and three of us speaking. Mark's brother Matthew spoke first and offered a deeply beautiful tribute to his brother. Kirk read what he had written about Mark saying many wonderful things, and ending with what has now become a beloved coined phrase for Mark as: *The man with a moral compass.*

Kirk then turned it over to me. After giving everyone a brief summary of our trip, and what an amazing impact it had on Mark from the moment we got there to the day he disappeared, I went on to say how special it was for both of us; all four of us, and how grateful I was to be with him for those last days and moments.

During the previous twenty-four hours I wrestled with what I was going to say at the wake. I wanted and needed to be free from my anger and eliminate the power from the darkness of it all. Instead of seeing the waves as haunting and taunting me for all those days, I thought, *You know what? I can turn it around. I have options. I can see it as this horrible evil or as a bright light behind it.* I needed for it to morph from an evil being into something beautiful in order to have closure, and to move forward with amazing memories of Mark deep inside our hearts as individuals and as a family.

I explained to the gathering of family and friends that, "I had originally thought of the set of waves as a horrendous evil entity crashing down upon Mark, but that now, instead, I imagine an amazing giant angel with big beautiful white wings coming behind him, and the arms of that angel wrapping around him and whisking him away to heaven. Mark wasn't able to choose how he died, but I guarantee you it would have been pretty close to how he lived—doing what he loved. The Lord threw us for a loop testing our faith as we wondered, hoped, and prayed during those five days. And on Sunday, we received a gift when Mark's body was found. It was nothing less than a miracle because we were told by some that he might never be found. The gift we received was closure. I'm grateful to the Lord for bringing Mark home understanding that this is much bigger than any of us. And a piece of Mark is hidden in each one of you. I see him. I feel him. I know he is here, and I'm grateful to God that he brought him home." I ended the service thanking everyone for their support and prayers.

When I told them a piece of Mark is hidden in each one of them, I meant whenever I see that person in the future, they will remind me of something different about Mark because of their special relationship with him. Friends and family are like flowers in a garden. They all offer different fragrances and textures, and it is the varied collection that makes a garden. In that way, our family and friends are not the same—the memories and moments are going to be distinct, but the garden remains melded together.

Upon our return home from the wake that evening around 9 pm, the four of us; Jacob, Lucas, Sami, and I walked into our house beautifully decorated with flowers and a huge spread of comfort food prepared and set out on our table with fine linens, flowers, candles, and wine. It was a surprise from two of my friends, Tina and Anna, who are Italian cousins of each other, and many years ago had adopted our family into their huge Italian family. Tina and her husband, Francesco, owned Nona Rosa's Italian Restaurant, and Anna with her husband, Gabby, own Donato's Floral, and Pickles Café and Catering, and all have been dug deeply into the Robbinsdale community for many years.

I hadn't eaten yet that day as I still had no appetite since Mark's disappearance. When I walked into our home and saw it transformed into a softly lit charming restaurant, and smelled the delicious aromas, I became suddenly hungry. Tina and Anna, along with other loving relatives and friends of theirs, served our children and me, and other family members, with a huge home cooked turkey dinner as if we were in a fine restaurant. It is a tradition in their family to honor a grieving family in this way instead of the family going to a restaurant after the wake. They first connected with my brother-in-law, Woody, to obtain a key to the house. While we were at the wake, they were at our house creating a cozy atmosphere with a delightful abundance of comfort food, knowing we'd be completely drained from the incredibly emotional and long day, and how nice it would be for us to be in our own home to breathe and feel safe. They stayed in the background and served us, and then graciously stayed to clean the dishes. They caressed us with their love and concern. What a merciful gift they offered to us.

I found out later from Anna that Jacob, Lucas, and Sami asked her how she knew turkey was their dad's favorite meal, and she told them she didn't know that. She said she herself finds comfort in a turkey dinner, and that pampering others with comfort food provides nourishment to a person's soul, and offers a little bit of normalcy after all the crying and tears that wreak havoc not only on our emotions, but on our body as a whole. Anna told me we can find beauty even in some of the hardest moments. That there is always something good.

And she got it right. In addition to pizza—chicken and turkey had been Mark's favorite foods. We were most certainly pampered and cared for.

NINETEEN

Mark's Funeral, Friday, March 8th

I dressed for the funeral and wore the amber necklace that Mark helped make for me on the beach our first day in Sayulita. It seemed so long ago. It was the last thing he ever bought for me, and certainly the only time he ever made jewelry for me.

I stood in our living room staring at the photo of Mark and me on our 25th wedding anniversary, a year-and-a-half earlier, when we renewed our vows. As I studied the photo and brushed my fingers across Mark's face, I realized that event would have been the last time many of those guests would have seen Mark since our vacation to Sayulita.

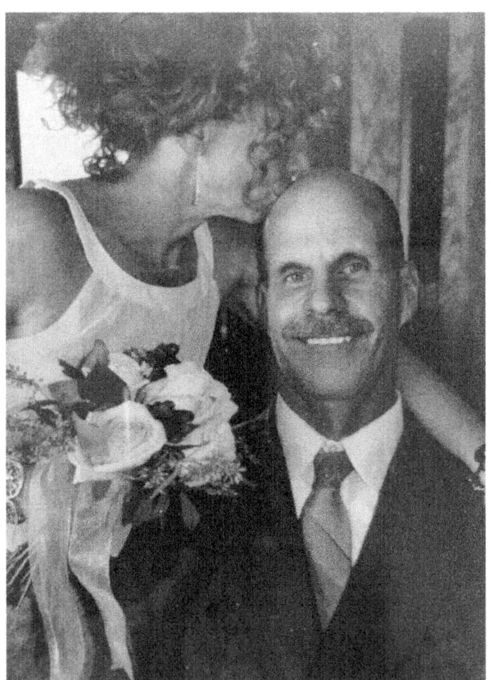

Our 25th Wedding Anniversary

I met with Father Pedersen before the Mass, and told him I didn't feel right sitting at the front of the church with my back to everybody throughout the entire service, other than when I processed in and processed out. Though I was able to talk to many people at the wake, there were others that I didn't get a chance to visit with. I felt the need to see people even within the extreme sadness and sorrow. I was heartbroken and in mourning, but I needed to speak because a miracle had occurred with Mark being found. My entire attitude could otherwise have been to forget the world and curse God. There was deep sadness, but there was also a silver lining in that God brought Mark back to us. I told Father Pedersen it was important for me, that if I had the strength, I wanted to be able to face the congregation if for no other reason than to look at them all and say thank you. I told him I didn't know if I could actually do it. I said I might be a puddle on the floor, but if I can, and if I only say thank you, it's what I need to do. Many of the people who were going to be there had supported my children when I was 2000 miles away; they were our community, and I just wanted to look at them and say thank you.

Father Pedersen suggested that when the time came during the Mass, when it was appropriate for me to come to the lectern, that he would look at me and I would nod yes or no. If it were yes, he would announce to the congregation that I wanted to say a few words to everyone.

Father Pedersen spoke about the insurmountable challenges we face in the midst of a life that appears to have been cut short, and the importance of leaning on our Lord as our rock and refuge in the midst of our grief—especially when things don't make sense to us. He discussed that when there is a tragic loss it is key to remember that even though God is with us on our earthly journey, there is a more critical concern about where we will spend eternity. He genuinely connected with our family in his eulogy telling many wonderful stories about Mark.

When the appropriate time came for me to address the congregation, I nodded yes. I reached the lectern and looked out at the completely filled, standing room only church. It was an overwhelming outpouring of love for Mark, me, my children, and the rest of our family. The first thing I said was, "Well, I guess we've certainly been thrown a curve ball, haven't we?" I said that because so many of our friends that we played ball with over the years, and Mark's friends and coworkers that he played many types of ball with, were in attendance. I wanted to honor those friendships and of course other friends and coworkers as well. Since Mark had been with Xcel for nearly forty years, his fellow linemen came out in droves to honor him.

I continued telling everyone, "The landscape of our journey has changed, but the destination remains the same. To live life to the fullest as we're not guaranteed tomorrow, and to always remember our Mark. It is different now. All of what I used to visualize, all of what my mind could possibly comprehend when I was in an especially good place, in a good world, with good people, and I looked forward to the next day, week, and ten and twenty years down the road, I could envision the future. More than seeing it, I could *feel* it. And then in an instant. Poof! It was gone. And now I struggle to think forward five minutes or longer. Because five minutes from now is not going to be the same as it was just a nanosecond ago.

"And it's not just about my Mark dying. It's about anyone who has loss and experienced pain. To me that is the craziest thing. It is the simplest things, the simple pleasures that we don't typically think about like drinking a cup of coffee the next day. It's not ever going to *taste* the same, and it's not going to *feel* the same drinking it anymore. It is that small. And it is that huge."

At the conclusion of the Mass, we invited the congregation to a luncheon at the church before processing to Gethsemane Cemetery about three miles away. A huge group gathered for the luncheon continuing the outpouring of affection for Mark, me, our children, and family. The room filled to overflowing with many standing and eating their food around the perimeter as there was no room left to sit. I mingled as much as possible before we needed to head to the cemetery.

The display of vehicles lined up to process to the cemetery profoundly humbled us. In an amazing and deeply heartfelt tribute to Mark, Xcel Energy cleaned and polished his truck, and it was included in the caravan. Mark's sister Missy told me that a friend of hers, who works for the detail shop that Xcel used, happened to be the person cleaning Mark's truck, and that she made extra efforts to make it shine exceptionally bright both inside and out. A co-worker of Mark's drove his truck in the procession, and it rode directly behind the family vehicles followed by numerous other Xcel trucks driven by his co-workers, with a tremendous line-up of family and friend's vehicles stretching a long distance behind.

Again, my children and I encouraged one another saying, "We can do this." We drove Mark's SUV and put another one of his CDs in the player and cranked up the volume; blasting it. It seemed like he was with us and encouraging us. It was spiritually powerful—and it was emotionally sad. It spanned the entire spectrum of emotions. We played Manowar's song "Warriors Of The World United."

> *Brothers everywhere*
> *Raise your hands into the air*
> *We're warriors*
> *Warriors of the world*
> *Like thunder from the sky*
> *Sworn to fight and die*
> *We're warriors*
> *Warriors of the world*

After the cemetery, a large group gathered at Broadway Pizza to continue celebrating Mark's life. That day, Xcel retired his truck. No one was allowed to drive it again.

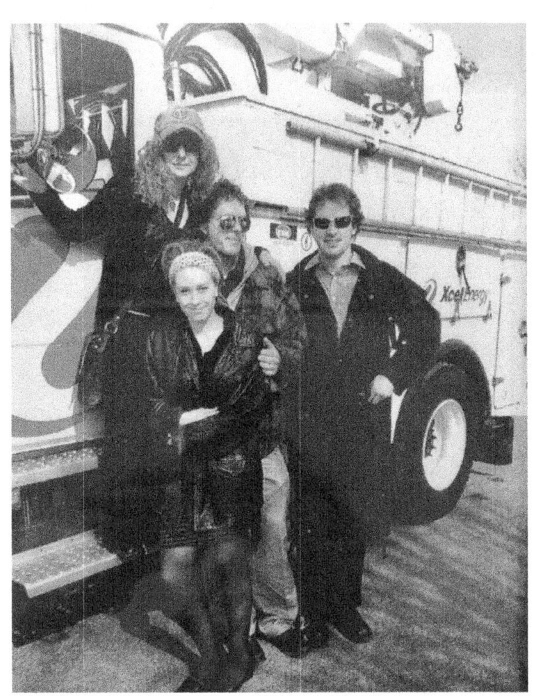

Me, Jacob, Sami, and Lucas

TWENTY

Moving Forward 'With'

For a long time after the funeral, my children and I continued receiving support and well wishes from friends and the community. Several days after the funeral, I read an article in our local Sun Post newspaper saying that the Robbinsdale City Council held a moment of silence for Mark and our family during their March 5th meeting—the same day I flew home from Mexico with Mark's ashes. In the article, the Robbinsdale mayor and council members stated how important it was to let me and my children know the community was thinking about us, that Mark was a beloved father and friend to many, that he was going to retire in June to enjoy the fruits of his labor, and that now those plans were cut short.

The only additions next to our family photo on the illuminated shelf in our living room hutch since Mark's passing is a memorial candle, a single photo of Mark, and four mini urns with his ashes. The large urn holding most of his ashes is at the cemetery in the mausoleum, and the four small ones are for me, my Jacob, my Lucas, and my Sami.

My sister Joanne came to my house every day for the first few weeks after Mark's death to keep me company, along with many different friends and family members who came over just to sit with me.

Both a Minnesota senator, and congressman at the time, called me to offer their condolences. The senator told me that he himself had experienced a terrifying experience with a near-drowning. I'm not sure what the extent of their involvement included with helping in the search effort, but I appreciated their sympathies.

Over the next few weeks, utility bills, phone bills, and other mailings started to arrive. I set them aside in a pile to look at later. Life still goes on and I was not ready for it. Businesses needed their money despite me mourning my husband's death. The person who was my heart and soul is now gone. But nothing else stopped. I had to try to be normal and pay the bills. Yet, I simply didn't have the energy to pay them. The task seemed insurmountable. Finally, when it came time to when I could no longer ignore the bills, I began opening the envelopes and paying them. When I opened the Verizon bill and saw a balance due of zero it confused me. I thought, *With all the calling and texting for several days, how could it possibly be zero?* I called Verizon and spoke to a representative. She said they wiped away the debt out of respect for our tragedy in losing Mark. *Wow.* Not only did they extend my usage while in Mexico, they zeroed out my balance completely. I had to catch my breath. I sincerely thanked the Verizon representative for their benevolence, hung up the phone, and stood staring at the zero-balance recalling those horrid days chalking up a huge phone bill in the effort to find *my* Mark, and staying in contact with my family and friends back home.

I lived in a deep fog for the first several weeks and months after the funeral, experiencing bouts of anxiety with my mind racing that seemed to come out of nowhere. It felt like my brain was struggling to rewire itself as it learned how to live without Mark after twenty-six years of marriage, and having been together since I was nineteen.

I am grateful that my children and I have a strong family and friends support network. The four of us worked together and separately through our individual grief. We didn't talk about the details of Mark's disappearance. The wound was still too raw. But we all knew we had our unspoken, unconditional love for one another, and that talking about it was always on the table.

Though we didn't talk about the tragedy in Mexico, we referenced Mark all the time. We still continually bring our Mark into conversations to keep him alive—*never* forgotten. Because how could we not? Mark was part of the fiber of our lives. Every moment of every day we simply couldn't have much of any conversation without him being part of it. And it's so beautiful. I know it is common that some people feel uncomfortable bringing up a deceased person's name to the survivors of their loved one, but we want the memory of Mark to be alive and present in our conversations. Always. It is *our* privilege.

A short while after the funeral, I ran into one of my clients from the club and she observed how much I spoke about Mark, and asked me if other people felt uncomfortable when I do so. I told her I didn't know, and that I hadn't thought about if it made others uncomfortable. She told me that after a brief time of mourning the death of her baby, when she mentioned her baby's name, it made people uncomfortable. She said she could feel the discomfort in the air, so she simply stopped talking about her baby. She told me how painful it was not to mention her baby's name, and my heart ached for her. For me, I don't care. I'll continue to talk and reminisce about *my,* Mark, *our* Mark, until the day I die.

I understand that there are reasons why people don't want to bring up a deceased person's name. One, because they think it will create more pain for the grieving person. Another, others determine in their mind what is a healthy amount of time to mourn, and after that it's time to 'move on' or just 'let it go.' There is no right or wrong way to mourn.

There is an author, Nora McInerny, who is known worldwide for her books and talks revealing her cathartic approach to loss and grief. She discusses a six-week period in her life, at age thirty-one, when she miscarried her second baby, lost her father to cancer, and became a widow when her husband died of brain cancer. Nora's common mantra: "We don't 'move on' from grief. We 'move forward' with it." I'm so grateful for her work and agree it's not about moving on 'without' but moving forward 'with.' She hits right to the core of grief and its deep trauma and does so with her gift of witty observational humor. She reminds me much of myself in that I can experience grief this way or experience it that way and I, like her, have chosen a positive alternative path. In one of her TED Talks she says, "A grieving person is going to laugh again and smile again. They're going to move forward. But that doesn't mean that they've moved on."

That first year my children and I strived to stay in the present. We learned how important it was to keep with tradition as much as possible in order to allow a sense of structure and security following Mark's death.

The first event that occurred after the funeral was to celebrate my birthday on March 17th, just ten days after the funeral. Someone suggested going to a local casino for the day, so about thirty of us took a shuttle bus there. I unfortunately don't remember a whole lot about that day.

The first holiday that followed was Easter on March 31st, just a little over three weeks since Mark's funeral. I asked my children if they wanted to stick with tradition and do our normal big celebration with an Easter egg hunt and food for about thirty to fifty people, or did they want to start a new tradition? I was fine either way. I wanted them to do what they wanted to do, and they unanimously agreed to keep it the same. So, we did with an empty aching in our hearts.

The next big event was Sami's prom a couple of weeks later. I bought her a beautiful dress and rented a limousine for her and her girlfriends. We had an all-afternoon pre-party at our house for the girls and some of the moms. I ordered in food. We listened to music and had a fun time helping the girls do their hair and get dressed, and then watched as they stepped into the limousine and drove away. It really was a fun day during such a sad time.

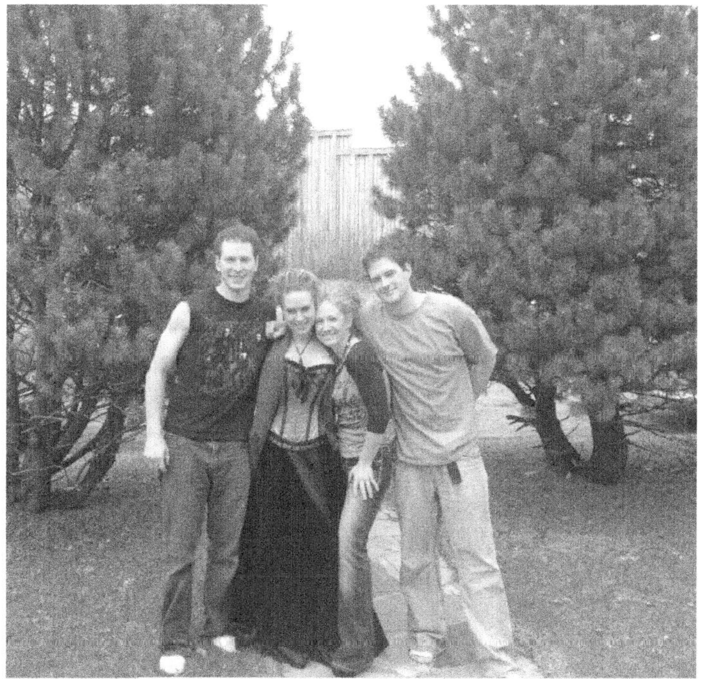

Sami's Prom: Lucas, Sami, Me, and Jacob

As time moved on, many of my family members and friends told me about Sami's strength during the torturous five days of Mark gone missing.

They said she kept her bearings; she was strong and steadfast. It had been excruciating for me that I couldn't be there *with* and *for* her, Jacob, and Lucas, and was grateful that she found ways to dig deep in order to keep it together with the strength of her brothers by her side.

Next, was Sami's high school graduation in early June. I asked her what she wanted to do to celebrate, and she said she wanted a party with a Jamaican theme. We threw a fully catered big bash with well over a hundred people that started in the afternoon and went into the evening. We decorated to the hilt. The Jamaican food was incredible; we had an amazing sound system playing great reggae music, and had a blast with a company-run photo booth who provided all kinds of props. It was a drizzly day, but it didn't matter as the yard was tented and it turned out to be a wonderful celebration despite Mark's absence. A bitter-sweet "fake it till you make it" effort for everyone. We mourned Mark's passing each and every day and celebrated his life within each event.

Then two weeks later would have been Mark's 59th birthday on June 21st, nearly four months after his death. Again, I asked my children what they wanted to do, and they said they wanted a party. So we had another party. We celebrated with much sorrow in our souls. It was difficult but it was necessary, and we hosted a huge barbeque, again, with over a hundred people, all offering toasts and sharing happy memories of Mark. If he had been alive, this birthday party would likely have been a combination of his official retirement party considering his age and time in service, as he started for Xcel on March 4, 1973. His body was found by the fishermen on March 3, 2013—one day short of 40 years to the day that he started at Xcel.

The day started out as a gorgeous sunny day that later turned stormy and rainy. Mark's birthday fell on the same day that severe rainfall, hail, and strong winds had caused widespread damage throughout Minneapolis and the surrounding suburbs. We were outside at first but moved the party inside as the storm grew stronger. It had been a historic deluge of rain that flooded some areas of our home as sheets of rain blew fiercely sideways pummeling our closed doors to the porch; penetrating through to the inside of our house. Nothing like that had ever happened to our house in the twenty plus years that we have owned it.

Mark's sister, Missy, had received a wonderful surprise at the party. Her son, Eric, asked her to come out to his car to show her something. She refused as she didn't want to run out into the torrential rain, but he insisted. She grabbed an umbrella, and when she got to the car, the passenger door opened, and it was their other son, Alex, whom she hadn't seen since his deployment to South Korea several months earlier. Alex was the son that couldn't get military leave to attend his uncle Mark's funeral. Missy threw down the umbrella and stood hugging him and sobbing joyous tears that commingled with her already rain-drenched face. Missy came back into the house with Alex in tow surprising the rest of us, and the party continued with mixed emotions of joy in seeing Alex, and sorrow in Mark's absence at his own birthday party.

The storm ravaged the metro area. Downed trees had crashed on top of power lines leaving nearly 100,000 residents without power, and flash flooding devastated homes making many roads impassable. Xcel Energy worked diligently for five days to replace over one hundred poles and thirty-seven miles of utility wires throughout the city, and they confirmed it was the largest power outage in company history. No doubt all of Mark's co-workers would've been tirelessly working overtime starting on his birthday, and he would've been officially retired that very same day. Mark likely would have reached out to Xcel Energy saying if there was an opportunity for him to come out of retirement to help with the repairs, that he would gladly assist. It would have been his last hurrah.

We woke to news the next morning that two blocks away from our house a water main had burst open on a major road creating a sinkhole fifty feet wide and twenty feet deep at the city's busiest intersection, and fortunately no one was hurt.

I thought about that day being historic and unusual with weather conditions of strong winds, rain, and flooding, and I couldn't help from paralleling the unusual weather conditions of wind and giant thunderous waters on the day that the waves took my Mark.

I moved slowly back into being mindful of my health by working out, trying to get enough sleep, and taking little power naps when needed.

I can doze for ten minutes and feel well rested. I have the gift of my father's napping ability. Growing up in Grand Forks, my dad used to come home for lunch. It was like clockwork. After my dad ate lunch, he laid on the couch falling asleep to Paul Harvey's light storytelling radio program, and when he heard Paul Harvey say his classic line, "And that's the *rest* of the story," my dad would pop up off the couch and go back to work after about ten minutes of shut eye.

When I owned It Figures, I got up every day at 4:30 am to open the club for the women, and by around 3:30 pm I would often go to my house a few blocks away, nap for ten minutes, and feel refreshed enough to go back to the club for a few more hours. I believe my ability to nap is what helped me in Sayulita. No rest during the day, with trivial sleep at night. I know the benefits of a good night's sleep, which I did not get there, and believe the cat naps were my saving grace. *Thanks for that gift, dad.*

I resumed my role as commissioner on the planning commission, as we only met once a month, and I handled that just fine. However, I did not resume training clients one-on-one right away. The one-on-one was so important for the benefit of my clients, but I didn't have the energy. I just could not do it. I could not even go through the motions to "fake it till I made it." I didn't possess the genuine vitality needed for that. I could have tried but I would have failed. Mark had always told me that when I smiled my eyes smiled too—that I had *smiling eyes*—and if I ever faked a smile, he would call me out on it. If we had to be somewhere around others and I wasn't feeling up to it, he would try to make me smile, and I would *put on* a smile. He would joke and say, "No. That right there? That smile? It's listed in the dictionary under fake smile."

I also didn't return to the "Twin Cities Live" TV show as their 'workout guru' for the same reasons—lack of vigor and exuberance. And the staff at "Twin Cities Live" had been so kind to me. They sent me a large portfolio of sympathy letters and cards which deeply blessed me, and informed me that when I was ready to come back, I was welcome any time.

While I wasn't up for doing training sessions for the TV audience, I did appear on the show several months later for an interview with the hosts, Steve and Elizabeth, to talk about the mourning process. It was a tough one. I almost lost it.

I didn't have smiling eyes to offer anyone at that point. But my women's group, the ones who I met with for Saturday morning bootcamp, who had a key to my house, who were with my children while I was in Sayulita; they started coming to my house immediately to work out in the gym, and I appreciated those relationships more than ever before. They would arrive around 5 am, and I would grab a cup of coffee and watch them work out, or sometimes even work out with them—they were my friends, my workout partners. They helped me make it through so much anguish. They were the reason for me to wake up and breathe because if they didn't come into the house, I know I wouldn't have gotten out of bed. I could have told them no. I had no desire or ambition to do anything, but they pretty much said, "Well, we're going to be here whether you like it or not. Mark would want us to be here, right? If all you do is sit with a cup of coffee in the gym that's fine. You don't have to say or do anything, just be here with us. We'll be here for you."

The year before Mark's death we had a local contractor draft a redesign of our main floor. The kitchen and living room were separated by a wall and the plan was to take down the wall to create an open concept. The plan was to have our house done and maintenance-free for the summer and fall, along with our maintenance-free townhome in Arizona for the winter. We didn't want to have projects in either place. It was all part of the retirement plan. I told Jacob, Lucas, and Sami that I wanted to cancel the redesign, but they encouraged me to move ahead saying it would be good to have something new for the house, and to follow through with the plans I had with their dad.

We started construction July 4th weekend. My friends continued to show up to work out. The main level of the house was gutted but my friends kept coming to work out in the basement gym. I had a full kitchen downstairs as well, so I could still function during the construction. It was about camaraderie. They had my back. Whether I wanted or needed them there, they were there no matter what. Five to six days a week they were at my door, and they had keys to my house, so even if I wasn't able to get out of bed because maybe I was in a dark place, which was fine, they were there for me. And if not all of them were there, most of them were. It was so very powerful and necessary even though I didn't fully realize it at the time.

That group of women loved Mark. When he was alive and we were all downstairs before he left for work, he would kiddingly holler down, "It sounds like a hen house down there! I hear too much cackling!" We would all laugh, and he would yell, "Get back to work!" And then he'd leave for the day.

Most of the remodeling had been completed by the last week in October with the completion date of October 31st—Halloween.

After we had celebrated Mark's birthday in June, and aside from the construction, the following four months had consisted of much down time for me psychologically. A few days before Halloween, Liz had asked me, with some hesitation, if I would be willing, wanting, and able to have a Halloween party for our family and friends which would be about a hundred people. At first, I thought, *What!* I didn't know if I was mentally up for it. Then after careful consideration, I decided with a spirited *why-the-hell-not* attitude—of course, what better way to really break in a remodel than to have a hundred people at the house! I agreed, but said I didn't want to prepare any food, so I put the word out that it was going to be a potluck, and let people know that I was going to be floating around the party and not playing hostess. I didn't know if I would have the ability to fully participate in the silliness essential for a costume party, and I needed a costume that would allow me to enjoy the party while staying in the background. In talking to one of my friends about a costume, we had an *aha* moment. We came up with the idea of me being a mime. It was brilliant. Since Mark's passing, I had grown used to not talking much, so the idea of being a mime seemed perfect. I created a few flip cards beforehand with some answers to anticipated basic questions, so that when someone asked me a question, I simply held up a response card.

The actual day of Halloween was on Thursday, but the party would happen the next night on Friday. The contractor was running a few days behind schedule in completing the renovation. When I explained to him about my plan for the party, he said they would have it all done by then.

On the morning of the party, the appliances were in my living room and the front steps weren't even built yet. The furniture was in the house but set off to the side. My friends showed up to work out and looked at me like I was insane. And I told them the contractor said it would all get done. It was like an HGTV hyper-drive deadline. The house buzzed with workers. I told them that people were coming whether it was done or not. They rose to the challenge and got everything completed with the exception of a pillar that I planned to have covered with stone, so they temporarily painted it instead. No one but me knew that was the only thing left undone.

With me dressed as a mime, my children wondered how long I could possibly go without talking as everyone knows I'm one who enjoys good conversation. Both the upstairs, downstairs, and outside patio spilled over with people in costume. I went downstairs for a bit and on my way back up I tripped, and someone yelled, "Are you okay?"

I yelled back, "Yep!" without realizing it. They caught me talking, but I quickly went back into the mode of being a mime and didn't say a word the rest of the evening.

There were so many great costumes that night, and Mark and I would have coordinated our costumes like we always did. Though he was a straightforward; highly disciplined man, he loved the frivolousness of costume parties. Jacob wore an Old Man mask, Lucas dressed as a keg of beer, and Sami, with her natural dread locks that she had been growing for a couple of years, made for a perfect Medusa. Mark's sister, Missy, dressed as a put-upon office worker and his sister, Donna, was a fully clad zombie.

And the remodel? I love the open concept with the kitchen that now flows into the new living room that Mark and I had designed together. I enjoy cooking, and the open concept allows me to cook and not have to miss out on socializing during gatherings, as compared to my old kitchen which was more closed off. The kitchen now has a granite countertop, but we saved the melted laminate piece with the hookah coal burn from our children's party—while we were in Mexico—as a reminder of how things like that do *not* matter within the reality of losing our Mark.

Even though we had kept with traditions since Mark's passing, because they had been ingrained in us over the years, in reality, the change for us individually and as a family of four had been tremendously difficult. We were moving on '*with.*' Over time we each started morphing into an altered identity apart from who we were with Mark, while perpetually keeping him close in our hearts. We each started to grow stronger and more resilient as time passed by.

Mark's sister, Missy, and her husband, Ken, moved in shortly after the remodeling was completed and stayed with us until they moved into their new home in December, 2013. They had lived about thirty minutes away and wanted to be closer to family. I let them stay in Mark's and my bedroom as I wasn't yet ready to sleep in there without him. The only thing that had changed during the remodeling in our bedroom was the paint color. The rest remained the same.

~~~~~~~~~~~~~~~~~~~~~~~~~~~~~~~~~~~~~~~

Striving to stay in the present proved more difficult than anything. My mind replayed the traumatic events that remained at the forefront of my thoughts. The reason our story had to be written is that I could not get it out of my mind. I feared that I would forget. And I'd ask myself, *Why did I not want to forget? Maybe I should want to forget.* I just had this horrible thought that there were things that needed to be remembered and the story needed to be told. I couldn't shut it down. Could not stop it. I would try. I would meditate, and the enjoyable times before Mark disappeared in the water to the calamity and hellish days afterward just kept playing over and over. Not the whole thing all at once, but bits and pieces that at times have driven me mad. Like that movie, *Groundhog Day*, playing over and over
~~~~~~~~~~~~~~~~~~~~~~~~~~~~~~~~~~~~~~~

and over again, but unlike the movie, I could not change the outcome. Something was telling me I needed to remember.

Whenever I've been out on a walk with someone and talking about losing Mark, my thoughts race and I get dizzy and have to stop and sit down. The myriad of thoughts of the entire seven days: The training we did beforehand. The suitcase full of food we slipped into the country. My first ever 'selfie' photo of the four of us on the private shuttle. Mark feeling the best he had felt in years. The treasured necklaces he helped make for me. Our first fairy-tale dinner at the skinny building. The kind bakery man and his son. The magnificent horse dancing. Surfing. The bottle bash game. Both the evil dogs on the roof at the festival, and the rogue dog that warmed up to Mark on the beach, and then later sat next to me at his beach memorial service. And as I thought more about the two evil dogs who maliciously stared and bared their teeth at us as we walked to the carnival on the day of the horse dancing—had they been a threat? A warning? Did they sense impending death in our presence? I will never know. But I will always wonder. I thought about the Irish pub and the whales breaching, and the Italian swing chair restaurant we planned to go to on the night Mark disappeared. Seeing the wave overtake Mark, and then desperately running up and down the beach. Dealing with the embassy and consulate. Sami's beautiful texts. Laying paralyzed in bed. David, the heroic search-and-rescue pilot. The military boat and identifying Mark's body. The wicked woman at the DA's office. Calling home and ripping off the band-aid. I thought about Liz's comment about me saving the man's life on the same day Mark lost his, and her asking why God would allow Mark to die. A good question for which I have no answer. I thought about the tender moment with the Delta pilot. But my thoughts are not in order as I've just described. They are jumbled in my mind and that's why I get dizzy. I've since learned that the dizziness is triggered as a symptom of Post-Traumatic Stress Syndrome (PTSD).

A few weeks after Mark's funeral I ran into a friend of mine at a store, and she broke into tears. I walked toward her and grabbed her hand. She asked, "Why? Why Mark?"

Tears welled, and I said, "Why not? Bad things happen to good people. Why is it that we rarely question the Lord or a Higher Power when good things happen to us? We receive it, we embrace it, we celebrate it. We don't question it. But when something bad happens we think *why me,* instead of why *not* me? Why would I or Mark be more special than anyone else in the world that has horror and tragedy present itself to them?" I said this to her not in a flippant way, but with a sense of resolve and I thought, *Why the hell not me? Why anybody?*

The next *first* holidays in 2013 without Mark were Thanksgiving and Christmas. We were all still on autopilot, and the children wanted to keep with tradition. We observed them both nearly the same as in previous years, but the only holiday I had anxiety about was the first Christmas. On Christmas Day morning, Mark and I and our children always did our little gift giving in the family room together with just the five of us. Then later in the day we celebrated with a larger family gathering. I wanted to move forward with this tradition but with a slight change. The only thing I changed without asking the children is that the gift giving was going to happen in the new living room, as I could not envision doing it in the family room without Mark. We began with a champagne toast to Mark with each one of us offering a special memory of him. And it has since remained a beautiful new tradition for us. After that, we enjoyed the rest of Christmas Day with the normal larger gathering of family.

TWENTY-ONE

Return To Sayulita For First Year Anniversary

In January 2014, I traveled to New York with some friends, and we went to a viewing area to look at the Statue of Liberty from across the bay. It was the first time that I'd been around big water since Mark had died, and I had a difficult time looking at the waves. It was a windy day, and all around us the water was quite active. Suddenly, my mind flashed back to those days and nights in Sayulita when I thought that Mark might have been floating in water similar to that. It bothered me a lot, and I told my friends that I just couldn't be out there.

Before the New York trip, I had already planned a trip to Sayulita with a large group of people to honor Mark's first-year- anniversary of his passing. I knew I needed to go back because as ugly of a situation that it was, it was still so beautiful to have been there with him those first four days, and I hoped there was going to be a connection to him there. I needed to feel that or at least see if it was there. I truly didn't have any idea how I'd feel, but I needed to go back and was willing to deal with whatever emotions were dealt. There was a draw—a need—to see what it was going to do to me. After the experience in New York, I was concerned as to what my reaction might be, but I needed to go. I presented the idea of going to Sayulita with Jacob, Lucas, and Sami along with other family members and friends, and said I was going no matter what and asked if they wanted to join me. I made it clear to everyone that the plan was to stay in Nuevo Vallarta and visit Sayulita just for the day on the anniversary of Mark's disappearance. I explained to them that I wanted to be at the place where Mark entered the water at exactly the same time he had entered, and to stay for two more hours until sunset. Jacob, Lucas, and Sami didn't hesitate. They, and the others who joined us, needed to see where Mark disappeared and all the places we had enjoyed the previous four days together. We stayed at our time-share in Nuevo Vallarta and being there didn't bother me a bit. A couple of days later, when we drove to Sayulita, it wasn't uncomfortable. I was fine. When we arrived in the Town Square, I stepped out of the shuttle and it was instant, there was a presence. It wasn't overwhelming, not painful, there was a connection and presence of *my* Mark, and I only felt the beautiful time with him. I never felt the ugliness.

We visited the area of the beach where Mark and Kirk had entered the water, and spent time at the northside of the beach at the rock memorial. Afterward, the couple who had let us use their computer for the vigil invited us to their camper where they offered us all a shot of tequila to toast to Mark.

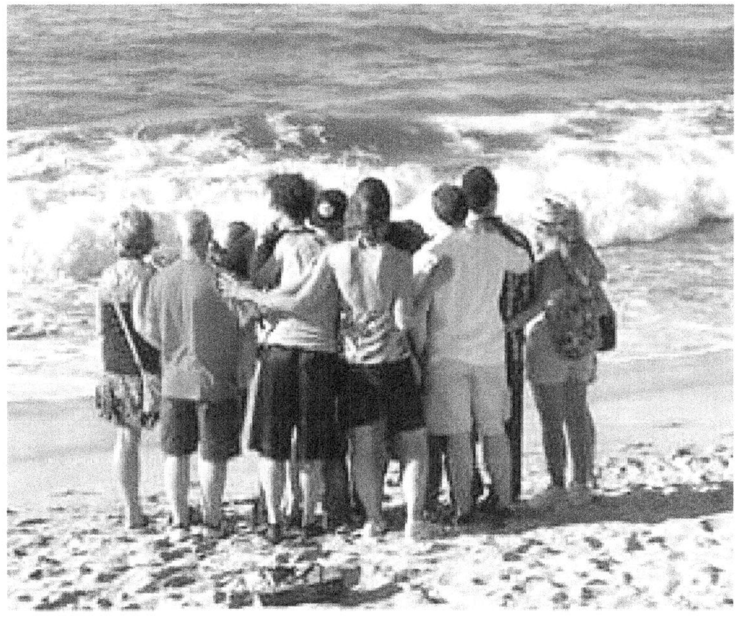

Family and friends standing where Mark and Kirk had entered the water.

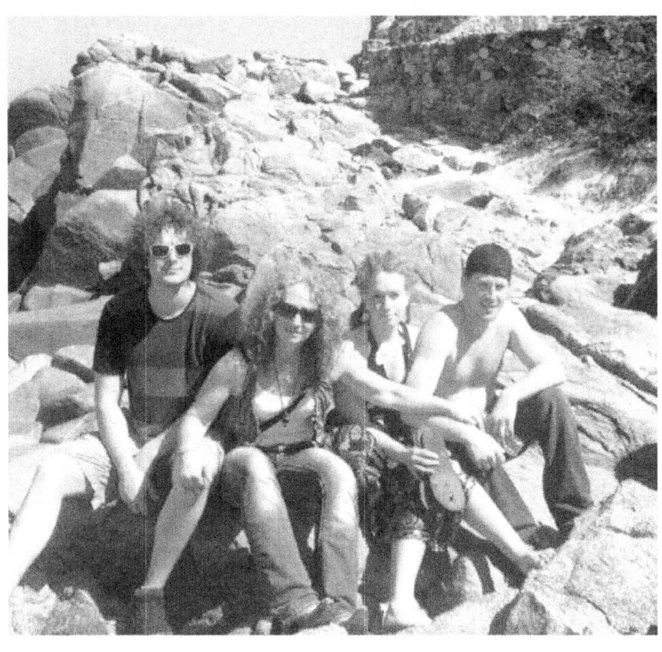

Jacob, Me, Sami, and Lucas at the northside beach memorial

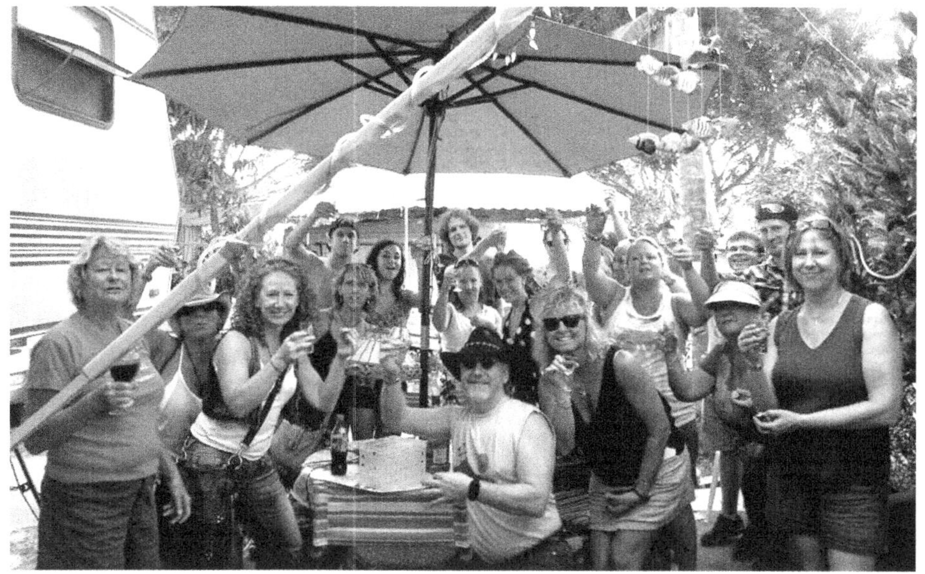

Patti, Me, Travis, Vicki, Courtney, Jacob, Maureen, Sami, Dave, Kathleen, Brian, Kim, Ivy, Patrick, Lucas, & Missy

That trip provided much healing for me and my children and other family members and friends. Despite the hue of the trip being tinged with various shades of gray, people were pleased to be there. We shared memories of Mark and created our own new ones.

The rest of the year, the second year, proved a little harder than the first year on some levels. The first year had been about survival and attempting to move on 'with' while trying to live within the routine of *the way things used to be*. The second year was more about stamina and searching inward. Who was I now that I was no longer part of a couple? Was I still a Misses or now a Miss? It felt strange when someone would call me Mrs. Stoneberg. That title seemed reserved for married people, but I didn't consider myself a Miss either. When filling out paperwork for the first time, and the form asked for my marital status, it felt abrasive to check the box for widow. Other times there wasn't a widow option on a form, and I had to mark single instead.

The support of the masses of people had lessened a bit, but I still had a strong support network with my children, my siblings, Mark's siblings, my girlfriends, and people in the community. My mom moved back into my house, and I had her stay in Mark's and my bedroom as I was still unable to sleep in there without him. I helped take care of her, along with my sister Joanne, who had become her primary caregiver as she continued struggling through Alzheimer's and other ailments. I continued going to church. I continued eating well and working out. Before Mark died, I'd always been the one to pay the bills, and we had a network of handymen to call when needed. I could still do many things, but I missed *my* Mark—my best friend and confidant. Mark would have loved the remodel that we designed together. The most difficult thing to deal with was the loss of intimacy with Mark and our future retirement dreams. I had always longed for us to grow old together.

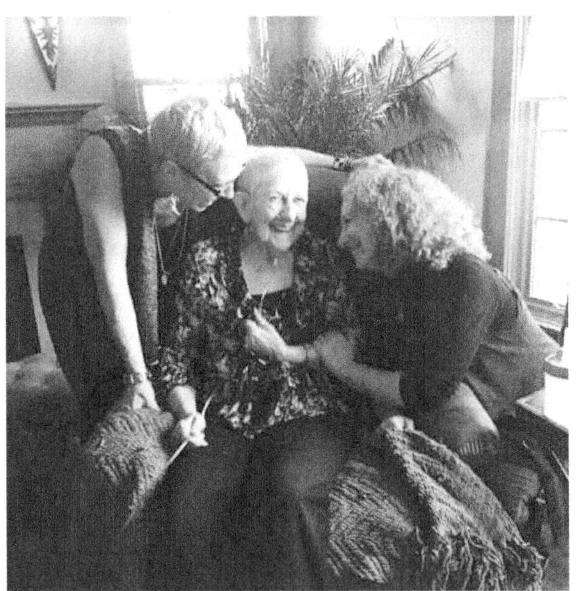

My sister Joanne, our mom, and me

In 2014, Kirk and Liz got married in Costa Rica. Kirk contacted me beforehand sincerely asking if he could borrow something that was special to Mark that he could carry in his pocket on his wedding day. That it would be an honor to have something of Mark's since he was to have been Kirk's best man. I gave him a tiny screwdriver that Mark kept on his key ring. It was very old and worn and had no doubt helped Mark many times over the years.

TWENTY-TWO

A Year of Fifty Firsts

After the first year, I was ready to start training clients one-on-one again. There was certainly sadness in my heart from losing Mark, but I missed working with my clients, so I started training others again. Nobody pressured me. Everyone was kind, and it felt good to be back with my clients in my home gym, and at a nearby senior condominium complex to continue my *empowerment* training with them.

In the spring of 2015, I resumed teaching religion classes at church to prepare children for their First Communion. On my first day back, I introduced myself to the class, and one of the young girls raised her hand and asked, "So, why did you go on that vacation anyway?" It was apparent she knew that Mark had died there.

Her question blindsided me. I thought, *What!* I back peddled a bit and then told a brief accounting of the tragedy that the students could understand at their level. I asked if any of them knew someone who had died, maybe grandma or grandpa. I took the opportunity to talk about loss and life, and turned the lesson into teaching about death and its sadness along with the beauty of sharing a life.

In 2015, I turned fifty. Mark and I had planned a trip to Ireland for my fiftieth birthday along with Jacob, Lucas, and Sami, while also spending a couple of days in Scotland so Mark could golf at one of their famous golf courses.

In fact, that's one of the things Mark and I had talked about on the airplane to Sayulita—going to Ireland and Scotland with our children. The only other places Mark wanted to travel to after retirement was Australia, and to Africa to go on a safari. That was it. Mark didn't have a desire to travel anywhere else, but was on board with me traveling to other countries with other people. His primary interest was to split time between Minnesota in the summer, and Arizona in the winter.

I couldn't bring myself to go to Ireland or Scotland without him, so instead I made a pact with myself and created a plan called, "A Year of Fifty Firsts," as in fifty things I had never done before and wanted to accomplish in the year of turning fifty. It was a collection of traveling, staying local, doing simple things and eating new foods; nothing too elaborate, and some rather silly. One of the silly new things I did was balance three golf balls on top of each other. It really is *a thing*, and Mark would have been proud. I posted all the new events on my Facebook page and ended up achieving my fifty firsts' goal that year. While I enjoyed the traveling and trying new things, I wished Mark could have experienced the same sights, sounds, tastes, and smells with me. Despite the ever-present hollowness of losing Mark, I continued moving forward with him deep in my heart.

At age fifty I also sketched out a fifteen-year plan that by age sixty-five, I would have traveled to, and done something noteworthy, in every state in the United States and one country per year. The plan was to travel whether or not anyone else joined me. The first year I was well on my way and had traveled to Arizona, Texas, the five New England states, and Italy. Though Mark had been to Arizona a few times, I never had.

All of our children were now on their own, so the timing seemed right for me to venture out on my own as well. Jacob still lives near me in his own home, and at that time Lucas and Sami along with my niece Courtney, Joanne's daughter, had moved to Austin, Texas.

That same year, very sadly and suddenly, my brother-in-law, Woody, passed away on August 11, 2015. He had worked for Xcel for 35 years, and like Mark, had been looking forward to retirement. Without Woody as my brother-in-law, I might never have met my Mark at the work softball game. Woody had been very influential in our lives, and very close to Jacob, Lucas, and Sami. He had been the first person people would call for help with all sorts of things, and always responded graciously and with a smile.

TWENTY-THREE

The Extraordinary & Unexpected Silver Lining In Mark's Drowning

On the fourth anniversary of Mark's death, I went back to Mexico with Jacob, Lucas, Sami, and about twelve other people and stayed in Nuevo Vallarta. We visited Sayulita for the day just as we had done on the first anniversary of Mark's death, and walked near the bungalow where Kirk, Liz, Mark, and I stayed four years prior. A gentleman recognized me and called out motioning for me to come over. He said he knew who I was and asked if I knew about the efforts happening to get a lifeguard stand on the northside of the beach. I told him no. He said the real change happened not only because Mark had drowned, because others unfortunately had drowned as well, but the five days of media exposure for Mark had stirred up an increased level of importance, and has been key to broadening the fundraising for life saving programs that others had already begun.

I had no idea. I got all goose pimply, "What?"

He said money had started funneling in from the family and friends of another man who drowned in 2010. He gave me the name of Janice Parker with Pro Sayulita, (aka Grupo Pro Sayulita), a local volunteer beach safety group comprised of snowbirds and natives, and then our group left to catch a shuttle back to Puerto Vallarta. I connected with Janice when I returned home, and she sent me the following message:

Hi Nancy,

I understand you visited Sayulita trailer park yesterday. I am a volunteer with Pro Sayulita and run the beach safety program. Subsequent to Mark's accident I was able to get the attention of Proteccion Civil, a government agency that runs lifeguard programs. We have been able to secure lifeguards here on this beach most days. I also run the volunteer lifeguard program in conjunction with Firefighters Crossing Borders (FFCB). We have annual training sessions here on the north side beach. To date we have trained about 100 volunteers. On the second anniversary of Mark's drowning, we had a very dramatic rescue of a woman in the exact same spot. Our lifeguards saved her. Last year on the very same date we had another rescue performed by our volunteers. We have named this rescue the 'Miracle Rescue.' The man had officially drowned and was out for more than twenty minutes. He was revived in the ambulance on his way to the clinic and is now leading a normal life with zero evidence of trauma. I just wanted to reach out and let you know this and tell you that although we did not know Mark he is forever in our memories.

After I read her message, I went on the Pro Sayulita Facebook page and found an old post from 2013 talking about the harsh weather season of 2011-2012 that had destroyed the signage that Pro Sayulita and FFCB had placed on the beach in the area where Mark had drowned. And that now, as a result of other lost lives, and because of the notoriety with Mark's drowning, the two groups were determined to continue warning people of the dangerous waters. After Mark's drowning they set up new flags and bilingual signs around the fragments of an old broken-down useless lifeguard stand on the north side. Back then, the group had started a type of neighborhood watch over the beach including volunteer lifeguards and patrols, and had purchased rescue boards. With those efforts alone about 150 rescues had been made by the end of the next season, and likely many more lives saved with people not entering the water at all because of the warning signs. I was completely unaware that this effort existed. Their post from 2013 makes it seem like there was a lifeguard tower at the time, but there were only the remnants of one from a long time ago, and it certainly wasn't occupied by any lifeguards.

I then looked in my Messenger account and saw that Janice had sent me a message way back on March 5, 2013. She sent a quick note letting me know how truly sorry they all were for our loss and included the poem, *Something Beautiful Remains*. Janice also said that she wanted to tell me about the beach safety project they had been working on there. I never saw her message until 2017.

The information about lives now being saved since Mark's drowning both gladdened and saddened me. I thought back to Mark's disappearance wondering if he could have been saved if lifeguards had been available, but then my mind quickly rushed to the scene of the tumultuous waves that early evening with no sight of him after the first wave crushed him, and realized Mark's drowning was an extremely rare one. My sorrow was mixed with appreciation for the other lives that have been saved, specifically because Mark and others had lost theirs. For me, it's not only about the number of lives that have been saved, as wonderful as that is, it's important that just one life has been saved. Because if you are the one they pulled out, or if you are the family of that one person, the impact of just one life has a huge rippling effect in and of itself. But then yes, of course, if you can multiply one human being by hundreds—it is a big deal.

I responded back to Janice, and she invited me back to Sayulita asking if I would tell my story about Mark's drowning at a fund raising gathering for the installation of the first of four planned guard towers starting in 2018. She said Mark's name, along with two other men who drowned in that area, would be on a plaque mounted to the tower. I jumped at the opportunity to be there and told her, "Absolutely, I will fly back and be part of the fundraising!"

I flew back three weeks later with a friend of mine and told of Mark's tragic story to the large crowd. I was elated to find out that they ended up raising enough money to move ahead with building the first guard tower— on the north side of the beach.

Janice had been part of the group that included the volunteers and firefighters back in 2013. I had no idea until 2017. When I was there for the fundraising, Janice told me she was on the beach almost immediately, and at one point behind me and embracing me on the night Mark disappeared. She was also the one who brought my blanket to me that I had left on the beach that same night. Though I have no recollection of Janice from that time, I'm so grateful *to* her and *for* her. And we have since become good friends.

I told my family and close friends about the commemoration that would happen the following year in 2018, and was so happy that many of them planned to join me.

I learned about the other men whose names were going to be on the guard tower plaque who drowned in the same area as Mark. They are Zach

Chambers, age 40, a US citizen who died on May 18, 2010, and Diego Ramos, a nearby Jalisco, Mexico resident, age 27, who died January 21, 2016. The date on the plaque for Mark is February 26, 2013, and I'm thankful that it's not the date on his death certificate of March 3, 2018, that the funeral director in Mexico insisted upon; so it means a lot that they are honoring the day that he disappeared.

In 2010, forty-year-old Zach Chambers died when on vacation with his wife and two young sons. At that time there were no lifeguards on the beaches of Sayulita, and Protection Civil y Bombero's was one hour away. Soon after his death, Zach's wife, and a good friend of Zach's with FFCB created the Zachary Chambers Sayulita-San Pancho Emergency Service Foundation. FFCB members are active and retired firefighters from Canada, the USA, and Mexico working to assist firefighters in Mexico. Over the years the FFCB, in cooperation with Pro Sayulita and Protection Civil, had trained dozens of volunteer lifeguards, and in 2014 the Zachary Chambers Foundation passed the torch to the local FFCB. Though there had been an increase in volunteer lifeguards, there was still a need for lifeguard towers, so the fundraising continued because the goal for Sayulita is to have four lifeguard towers along the beach. I'm grateful for the efforts of so many folks including Zach's wife, Pro Sayulita, the FFCB, and Protection Civil, that have resulted in the construction of the first tower on the northside honoring Mark, Zach, and Diego.

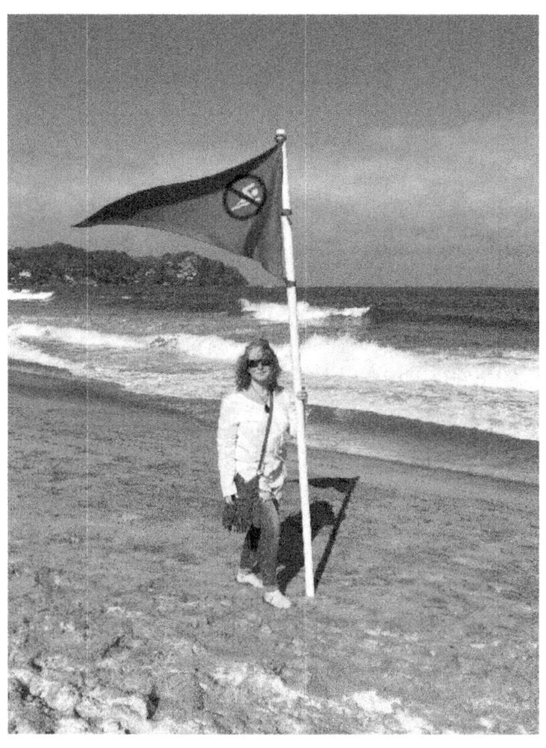

Me holding a warning flag on the north side of the beach in Sayulita

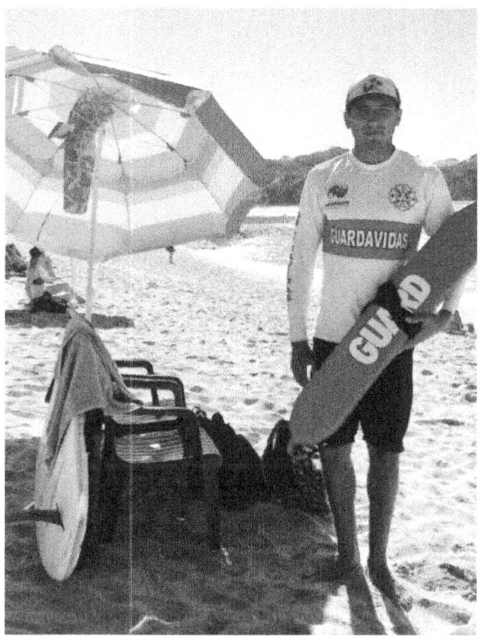

Volunteer lifeguard station before the installation of the first permanent lifeguard tower.

TWENTY-FOUR

Five-Year Memorial and Lifeguard Tower Dedication

In January 2018, I had written to Janice telling her that I would be attending the lifeguard tower commemoration with nineteen family members and friends, and the date we were arriving.

Unlike the other two visits when we stayed in Nuevo Vallarta and made a day trip to Sayulita, this time we planned to stay in Sayulita. I rented a house on the beach for the older people like me only two houses away from the bungalow where Kirk, Liz, Mark, and I had stayed, and another house down the block for the younger people.

Janice sent me another message on Messenger on February 19, 2018.

Good morning Nancy, thanks for sharing the article about Mark. I just want to clarify one thing so that you are aware of how this has worked. The Mexican government has not given us any money toward beach safety. We have raised 100% of the money by donations and t-shirt sales. The government in fact has pulled lifeguards once again. We sporadically have guards on our beach which makes our auxiliary lifeguard program all that more important. We are planning the dedication on Monday, February 26, 2018, at 5 pm at the tower which is located in front of the rip where Mark went missing. See you on Saturday. I will have your t-shirts at my casita.

Then on February 8, 2018, Janice, with Grupo Pro Sayulita, publicized the commemoration on the group's Facebook page about the new lifeguard tower on the north beach at the end of the street called, Calle Miramar, which is very close to the bungalow and only yards away from where Mark vanished in the ocean. The post included gratitude for all those who gave of their money and time to create a safe beach experience for both locals and vacationers.

I called my friends at KSTP-TV news to inform them of the good news, and they aired the story about a new lifeguard tower honoring Mark that would save lives even though he tragically lost his, and quoted me saying, "You cannot imagine the helplessness when all of a sudden there's an emergency and you're yelling and there's nobody to respond because help is simply not there." And about the lifeguard tower, I said, "Typically, there's not a silver lining. I'm very proud, and very sad."

On Friday, February 23, 2018, Grupo Pro Sayulita graciously announced the arrival of me and my nineteen family members and friends who would be arriving the next day to celebrate the lifeguard tower ceremony on Monday, February 26, 2018.

Some things had changed over the previous five years in Sayulita since Mark's disappearance with a rise in population of about 70%, and in my opinion the best change was the construction of the first lifeguard tower. Our group of nineteen hung out together, and also fanned out in different directions throughout the days and nights on Saturday and Sunday, and again on Monday before the scheduled ceremony at 5:00 pm.

On Monday morning, I sat with family and friends having coffee at a shop a couple doors down from the house we rented, and Sami was in the village with her cousin, Courtney. Sami was standing in the square when two men carrying a massive stunning floral wreath on top of a miniature surfboard walked by her and Courtney, and as she looked more closely, she saw part of a word *ERG* that caught her eye written on the large white ribbon placed across the wreath. She moved closer and saw that the ribbon read, *IN MEMORY OF MARK STONEBERG.* It deeply overwhelmed her to not only see her dad's name, but also on such a gorgeous and immense bouquet being paraded right next to her. She called to tell me about it right away, and as we talked for several minutes something caught my peripheral vision. I looked over my right shoulder, *Oh my gosh, there they are.* Chills ran throughout my body. I watched as the two men carried the wreath toward the coffee shop—one in front and the other following behind. The timing was bizarre. Sami didn't know that I was at the coffee shop or where the men were heading. I told her, "Baby, you wouldn't believe it, but they're right in front of me now." I stood up and saw that one of the men was Janice's husband and I called out to him. He looked over, and I snapped a picture of them with Janice's husband offering a compassionate thumbs up as they kept on walking toward the beach.

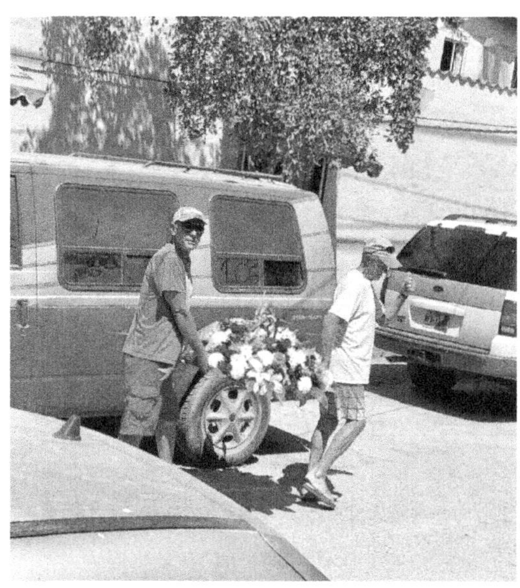

Men carrying Mark's memorial bouquet.

Right before the start of the dedication Janice approached me saying that twenty minutes prior, a woman had been taken by a rip and went under water, and that one of the lifeguards recovered her and ultimately revived her. When she came to, she was extremely distraught and told Janice she was helpless and struggling in the water and believed she was going to drown when she went under for the last time. After the woman had gathered herself, Janice told her about the ceremony that was going to happen in the next few minutes, and that she had been saved because of all that is now happening with lifeguards, and invited her to join the ceremony. The woman was grateful, but too upset and said she wouldn't be able to participate.

A local man, Jack Jones, opened the ceremony welcoming all attendees as a group of local musicians provided background music. The dedication started and Brian Singleton of FFCB, and Citali Darany Lopez Souza from Proteccion Civil, spoke about the commitment of the government to the Beach Safety Program, and that together with Pro Sayulita funding, would continue to build three more towers. Gratitude was given to Cyd Viator of Phoenix, Arizona, who built the tower himself out of 100% rot and corrosion resistant recycled plastic material that housed a special plaque including the names of Mark, Zach, and Diego.

As part of Huichol tradition, Oodette Gordon lit copal incense to cleanse the tower of any negative energy. Janice and I unveiled the inscribed plaque with Mark, Zach and Diego's names, and Janice read the following poem.

Something Beautiful Remains

The tide recedes but leaves behind
Bright seashells on the sand.

The sun goes down but gentle warmth
Still lingers on the land.

The music stops and yet it lingers on
In sweet refrain.

For every joy that passes
Something beautiful remains.
-Unkown

After the ceremony, a local man, Mark Rupert, led a traditional memorial paddle-out in Mark's memory. A paddle-out is a spiritual ceremony within the surf culture. For Mark's ceremony, many surfers paddled out on their boards, with one board carrying the glorious floral wreath. It was extremely moving. After the surfers paddled out beyond the break, they all joined hands to form a floating circle and chanted and sang in honor of Mark. They released the flowers, and the surfers all splashed the water to disperse them further out to sea.

The entire ceremony moved us in profoundly emotional ways—like a second funeral for Mark. And it provided Sayulita closure for me, Jacob,

Lucas, and Sami, as well as the rest of our family and friends, with the lifeguard tower and compassionate surfer memorial ritual.

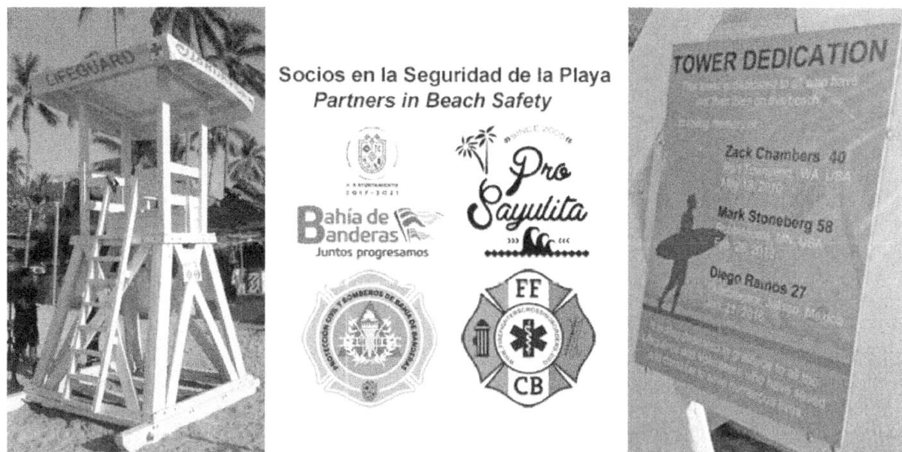

Lifeguard tower. Partners in beach safety. List of names on the tower: Zach, Mark and Diego.

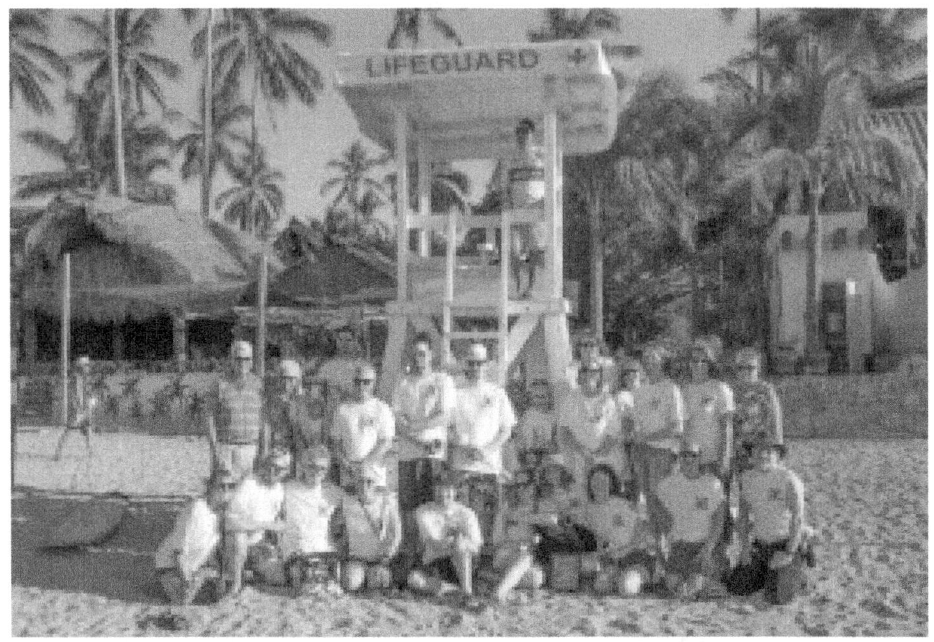

Family and friends in front of the new lifeguard tower

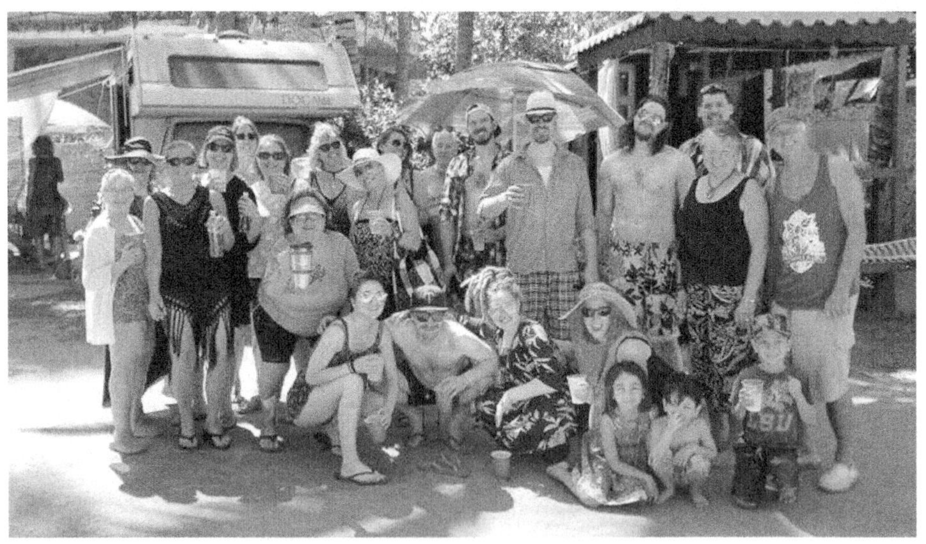

Family and friends at the trailer park

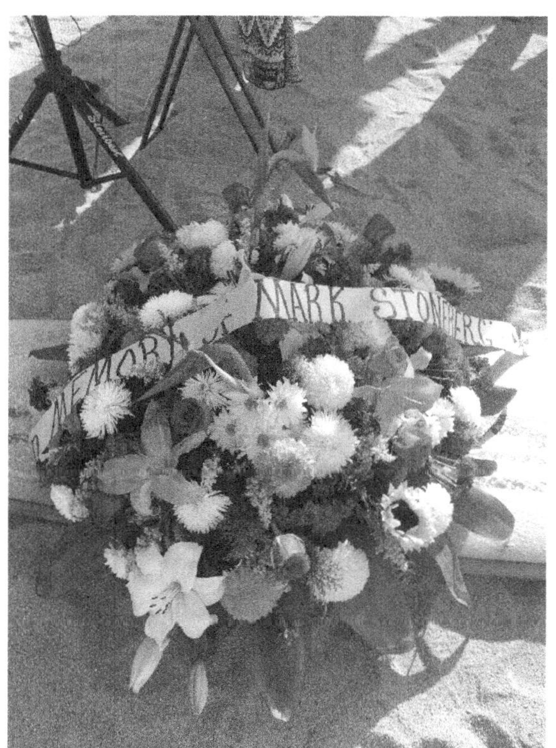

Mark's Memorial Bouquet

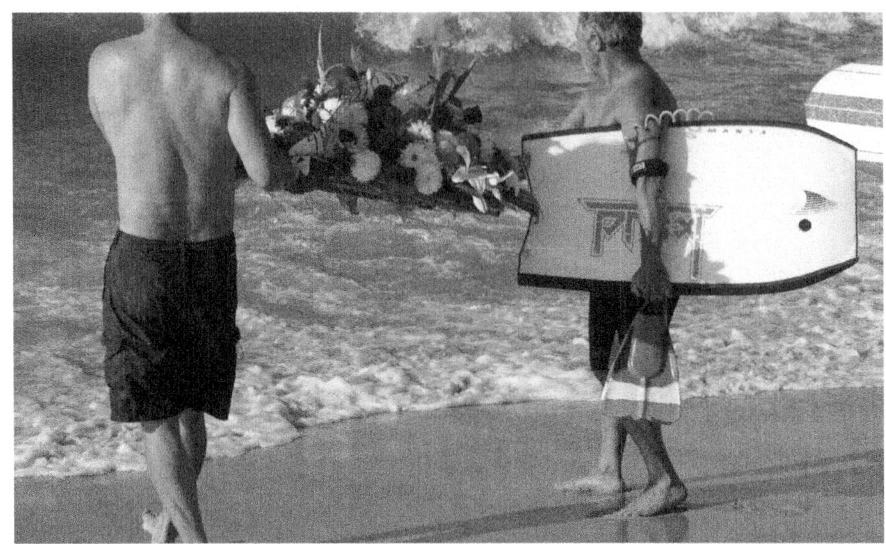

Paddle-out for Mark.

After the ceremony, people in our group scattered in different directions doing their own things. The annual carnival had ended two days before, but there were always outdoor activities happening in the plaza and around town. I relaxed at the bungalow for a bit and then walked into town with my friend, Lisa, to shop and meander around before sunset.

We stayed for a while and when it started getting dark, Lisa and I headed back to the bungalow. Jacob and my brother-in-law, Brian, saw Lisa and me and caught up to us. We turned down a little dirt road and came upon a beer bottle bash game. I stopped. Jacob turned to me with a knowing smile. I had previously told Jacob, Lucas, and Sami about the beer bottle bash game that their dad had played on our second night in Sayulita, and that not only did their talented softball throwing dad not break any of the bottles, but his first throw didn't even make it near the bottles. Jacob told me he had found a similar game earlier in the day near the plaza, and had spent a lot of money throwing and trying to break a bottle, but he also never did. Well, of course we had to play the roadside game in honor of his dad. Jacob tried again spending more and more money without success— just like his dad. I spent plenty of money without breaking a bottle either. It really is hard to break a bottle. It sits on a stick peg and just spins if you don't hit it just right.

Then, with one more rock left in my hand, I threw it, and lo and behold…it shattered the bottle. Jacob yelled, "You did it mom! Someone finally did it! Dad couldn't do it! I couldn't do it!" Jacob grabbed me, and we hugged. It was so very emotional. It seemed like a turning point for him after five long years in losing his dad and best friend. Almost as if it were dad making sure mom broke the bottle. It was a significant moment for both of us. The two of us strode arm and arm back to the house with Lisa and Brian, and the moments on our walk felt precious beyond words.

EPILOGUE

Nothing Less Than A Miracle

In 2019, I finally moved into the bedroom that I'd shared with *my* Mark during our twenty-six years of marriage. It had been remodeled with one closet expanded and another converted into a bathroom, and the walls had been painted a different color, so it didn't feel exactly the same, but it was still our bedroom, and the first night I tossed and turned as I hugged Mark's pillow for the first time since his passing.

Originally, I wanted the title of our journey to be, *Nothing Less Than A Miracle*, but we found that there are other books on the market with nearly the same title. As I thought more about the most fitting title, it dawned on me that since most people outside of our family called Mark 'Stoney,' it became the obvious choice. With that said, I still believe it is a miracle story—including not one miracle, but three.

Typically, miracles are *not* associated with a tragedy. One definition of a miracle I found is:

1. *A surprising and welcome event that is not explicable by natural or scientific laws and is therefore considered to be the work of a divine agency.*

Using the word miracle, whether in real life or fiction, always seems to relate to some kind of happy ending. The purpose for this story is to express that often-times miracles present themselves in different ways.

The first miracle in our journey is found in the events that transpired in the months and days before Sayulita. The opportunities that presented themselves with Jacob and Lucas spending much time with their dad playing softball and other things, the shift in the father and teen daughter relationship with Sami's boot shopping, Sami's letters home thanking him for those boots, the New Year's Eve party, our family together the night before we left on the trip, Mark and me on the airplane planning for our future, and Mark waking up pain-free every day in Sayulita. Collectively, all those things together were a gift from God—things that had never happened before, and that ended up being near the time of his death.

I believe miracles—the working of God on our behalf—happen every day that I don't see as miraculous at the time. Not necessarily the big shock and awe phenomenon's that happen outside of us, but in the daily mysteries we encounter. And when I take time to reflect daily and then retrace my steps, I see them and think, *Oh my gosh, there's another one.*

The second miracle is in finding Mark's body at all, as we were told the odds of finding someone taken out to sea in that area are extremely rare because it is the open ocean, not a bay. The locals had told us during those several days of searching that if a body didn't wash ashore after two days, it would never wash ashore.

And though it's certainly not a happy ending, the third miracle through losing Mark, is his legacy and the frequent saving of lives in Sayulita now and into the future with the construction of the lifeguard tower.

These are certainly three significant miracles and I've had to look beyond myself to be able to see that. I have to say that until the lifeguard tower was built, that Mark's death always felt bad. And I never want to ever feel that pain again. *Never.* It was bad with a bad ending. And it is still bad because Mark is not alive to be with us to experience all that life would have offered us as a family growing older together—and as a couple—continuing to change with age alongside one another. But now, because of Mark's death, and the subsequent tower and lifeguards, along with the warning signs, that people might be more careful and aware to not even enter the water in that area.

Unfortunately, often it is tragedy that begets change for a greater good. Not only did the story need to get out of my head and on paper because of the horrifying experiences of those days swirling in my mind, but that Mark's death ended up having a silver lining with lives being saved. And I say that with an aggrieved, humbled, and grateful heart knowing many sudden deaths do not have a silver lining for loved ones left behind. We all have either experienced, or know people who have experienced, the tragedy of losing someone before their time, and are left with painful, residual feelings of a bad death with no silver lining, and many unanswered questions.

I also realize that even though the lifeguards in the towers are saving lives, that there still remains much solace and grief for me, Jacob, Lucas, Sami, Mark's siblings, and other loved ones and friends.

A silver lining is only that. It is a veneer covering a damaged and heartbroken spirit. But a silver lining is meant to offer hope. I believe this earth is not our permanent home. And the hope we now have in losing Mark is believing we will someday be reunited with him to live peacefully and pain-free in heaven.

I believe if an angel had come to Mark in the water and that angel said to him, "Here's the deal. You can live, but I can't guarantee you will live even another week, and I can pull you out of this situation, or...you can allow me to take you right now guaranteeing there will be many, many lives saved because of your death." I know darn well that Mark felt fulfilled enough in his life and without a doubt he would have agreed to be taken saying to the angel, "Well, yeah."

We're all going to die. But how do we want to die? I would be honored to have my death be the outcome in saving other people's lives. Mark died doing what he loved and now lives are being saved as a result. It's terrible for those of us left behind, but to be able to die doing what you love is a gift. Mark did not get to say good-bye. I hate that Mark died, but we had a beautiful life with him, and we cherish every memory of him forever in our hearts.

Now, because of this awful tragedy in losing Mark, I tell others that when they travel to another country to be sure that they have the phone numbers of the closest embassy or consulate to where they're staying. That it's even a good idea to register your trip beforehand, so you can contact them if you have an emergency, and they can send you the latest information affecting US citizens in the area of a natural disaster or some other emergency.

I've visited the ocean many times since losing Mark. The beaches I've gone to have had calm waves and I'm okay being in that quieter environment. I don't know what it would be like for me if I were around thunderous waves like we experienced with Mark's drowning. But I've been at peace with the water in Sayulita because of the silver lining with lives being saved, and the waves haven't been tumultuous when I've visited there.

That said, I'm intrinsically aware of rip currents and knowing what to look for when I do swim in the ocean. I will only go to a beach that is familiar to me or to the people I am with. I have no interest in going to an uncharted beach on a secluded island somewhere. That thought terrifies me. I will no longer swim in the ocean at night as I had done previously in my life, and wouldn't be able to be around anyone else doing it either—I would have to walk away. When I see children in the ocean, I now look at that differently as well.

I admit I've been less than complimentary toward the Mexican government for the deficient emergency services and less than compassionate handling of our dire circumstances, but also realize we were in a small fishing and surf village. We had little knowledge of any behind-the-scenes activity and only saw the wonderful, dedicated locals like Janice, along with other Pro Sayulita volunteers and FFCB, who diligently assisted every day in searching by walking the beach and using the equipment that they had at their disposal—paddle boards in the water as they looked downward at the sea.

Upon further investigation, we found news articles stating that the year 2013 had experienced the most extreme and disordered weather events in decades around the world with record rainstorms, cyclones, flooding, and heatwaves. Perhaps that's why the waves were wickedly violent that day. We can't be sure. What we feel certain of, however, is that had the giant wave and two subsequent waves not crashed directly down on Mark that day, he would've been able to swim out of the rip current that moved him so quickly further out to sea. There are ways to successfully get out of a rip and Mark would have known how to do that. Rip currents don't bring you under the water, they just pull you away from the shore. He would have either allowed the current to bring him back to shore, or he would've swum parallel to the shore to get out of it because rips are narrow—only about 30 feet wide. But he didn't have a chance to do that. We believe that since

Mark didn't surface at all after the first giant wave forcefully hit him, that he possibly broke his neck upon impact. As awful as that is to imagine, it brings a sense of peace knowing it was instant.

Bonnie told me that during her research for the book she became curious about the significance of the numbers 3 3 2013 in reference to March 3, 2013, which was the morning Mark visited me on the day his body was found. The first thing that appeared on the internet was an excerpt from the International Electrotechnical Commission webstore as follows:

"IEC 61000-3-3:2013 is concerned with the limitation of voltage fluctuations and flicker impressed on the public low-voltage system. It specifies limits of voltage changes…"

Though Mark worked with public high-voltage versus low-voltage systems, we both found the correlation meaningful enough to ponder. And upon further research of the numbers 3 3 2013, Bonnie found something else interesting. It is from the Gospel of Mark.

Mark 3:13, "And He (Jesus) went up on the mountain and called to Him those He Himself wanted. And they came to Him." NKJV

While the gospel writer, Mark, had not been one of the original twelve disciples in this scripture verse, he became an eager follower, an apostle, who wrote about Jesus' ministry and servanthood. Again, we found this verse intriguing and don't ascribe any meaning to this verse or the voltage fluctuations beyond simply thoughts to contemplate considering Mark's name, his occupation, and his reputation as, "The man with a moral compass."

On February 26, 2021, I received the following beautiful tribute to Mark from Janice Parker. Janice continues to update the Pro Sayulita website lovingly remembering our Mark and others who had drowned, as well as those who have since been saved as a result of the lifeguard tower and increasing numbers of volunteer lifeguards. She and all the Pro

Sayulita members are unwavering warriors in the tireless pursuit to keep the beaches of Sayulita safe for residents and visitors.

Today marks the 8th anniversary of the drowning of Mark Stoneberg of Robbinsdale, Minnesota. Mark was here with his wife and another couple on Marks first surf trip. The sea was very rough that day and the riptide was super strong. At that time, the Northside beach had no signage and no lifeguard. Mark was swept out faster than anyone could get to him and unfortunately, he lost his life. However, this tragic event brought civic awareness to the dangers on the Northside. Our Sayulita Surf Rescue/Beach Safety Program was born from this event. Three years ago today, we dedicated our first Lifeguard tower on the Northside beach in honor of Zach Chambers, Mark Stoneberg and Diego Ramos who all lost their lives on this beach.

Today also marks the 7th anniversary of Sandra's rescue. Her "Re-birthday." Sandra took her last breath, said goodbye to her family in her mind and was going down for the last time, when Epsilon from Sayulita Surf Co. grabbed her and pulled her up from sinking. Sandra later told me that she felt like she was going up to heaven and didn't realize she had been saved until she was sitting on the beach.

Also, on this day 5 years ago, Geovani Perez of Sayulita Surf Co. brought Steve back to life after he had technically drowned. Happy "Re-birthday" to Steve!

Geovani has been very active in our Surf Rescue Program, not only in support of the program but also being very active in the training sessions. Unfortunately, due to COVID -19, we have been unable to schedule trainings for the past two seasons.

I would like to take this opportunity to thank each and every one of you who have taken our courses over the past years and who almost daily risk their lives to save others. Thankfully, there are many volunteers still in town. Hopefully soon we will be able to host more trainings and continue to educate our locals to help save lives and make our beaches safer places in which to play.

RIP Mark Stoneberg. You have helped us shape a program that works! Happy "Re-Birthday" Sandra and Steve.

SIDE STORIES

Heartfelt Testimonials Of Those In Sayulita And Others At
Home During Mark's Disappearance

Once again, my dear friend Janice with Pro Sayulita faithfully posted on their website on February 27, 2020, honoring the seventh anniversary of Mark's drowning on the 26th, saying his death and the subsequent safety program they have developed over the years continues to save more and more lives, and that they were working on another training session. She ended the post saying, "Be careful out there today. It's a rough one!"

Over a period of several months since our first session together in September 2019, Bonnie and I had captured the core essentials of our journey from my perspective, and I have received much healing in the process. But I remained haunted by some missing pieces that I knew others could provide to me, and hoped others would want to share their experience, not only for my benefit, but for theirs as well. Thankfully, some family members and friends agreed to share their memories of those tragic days.

Starting in June 2020 and ending in September 2020, Bonnie and I met with Dave and Patti, and Liz of Liz and Kirk, regarding their experiences in Sayulita, as well as my daughter Sami, Mark's sisters Missy and Donna, my sister Joanne, and my friend Kim with her husband Joe, who were all back home during those days and nights in 2013. I had also connected over the phone in December 2020 with the Delta pilot, Rob Reed, who had flown me home from Sayulita. I, unfortunately, do not have David the search pilot's contact information, though I wish I did in order to thank him again, and tell him of the resulting silver lining with the continuing safety program and lifeguard towers in Sayulita in part due to Mark's loss of life.

~~~~~From Dave and Patti: June 2020~~~~

Bonnie and I met with Dave and Patti in their home on a warm summer evening. They live just across the road from me and the four of us settled in their living room.

They both spoke nearly finishing each other's sentences as they remembered those dreadful days and nights in Sayulita.

To this day neither of them like going to a beach and listening to the ocean because they now find it haunting knowing that the ocean took Mark. Dave said the four nights of listening to the crashing surf and hoping for Mark's return ruined it for him. Dave said though it has been years, it feels like yesterday. That when he hears the sound of waves, he recalls lying sleepless on the cement bench every night expecting Mark to walk up at any moment, seeing him lying there, and asking him what he was doing there and questioning why he was worried.

Dave and Patti said what they remember most about being in Sayulita is the trauma. Dave said that he doesn't recall the specifics of going into town or conversations. He might remember if people bring up a situation, but it will always be the trauma. The trauma in searching. The trauma in not finding Mark. The trauma in identifying his body on the boat. The trauma at the DA's office with the armed guards standing over them, and the funeral home in Sayulita. Primarily—the trauma.

~~~~~*From Sami: July 2020*~~~~~

Bonnie and I met with Sami in a three-way phone conversation with the two of us each in our own homes in Robbinsdale, and Sami in her home in Oregon.

I asked Sami to just tell her story. She started with the night before we left for Sayulita at her cousin Trevor's farewell party. She said the party was a great send off for him leaving for the Guard, and everyone was just hanging out having a fun time, and that the five of us as a family were good together. She remembers getting dropped off at her girlfriend's house and saying I love you to Mark and me, and that the night felt really great.

She described herself at that time as an independent teenager hanging out with friends, not thinking too much about mom or dad because she didn't need to, and didn't want to as we were 'her parents.' But the night of Trevor's party, she said she appreciated being together as a family having fun while her dad happily doled out the money for the arcade games that we all played as a five-some.

Sami spoke about the 'stellar party,' as she put it, at the house that she, Jacob, and Lucas had on our first night away on Saturday and waking up the next morning seeing the square inch hole in the countertop from the hookah coal. She said they all thought it was the end of the world. They called Joe, one of Lucas's friends, to see if he could repair it, but he said there was no way to repair it without obvious signs of the repairs. They gave up on the idea of repairing it and decided they were just going to tell Mark and me what happened when we got home from Mexico. So, for three days Sami said they were extremely stressed about the hole, until clearly, that burn hole did *not* matter anymore once Lucas got the call from me.

Sami said she was in our bedroom doing her hair when Lucas came in with tears in his eyes telling her that dad was dead. Sami said at that moment her emotions shut off—she went numb and doesn't remember much after that.

I told her Lucas must have been in shock and confused at what he had heard from me, because I didn't tell him their dad was dead. She agreed saying Lucas really didn't know that at the time, because it wasn't until five days later that their dad's death was confirmed.

I asked her if she remembers talking to Lucas and asking him more about the phone conversation. She said she didn't press Lucas further, because evidently something bad had happened and she didn't want to be the one pushing. So she resigned herself to play the waiting game to hear more from me.

Sami said the five days at the house blended together. Every day, people brought over food and stayed around expressing concern for us, and that it was a heartfelt outpouring of support. She said the house filled nonstop with people everywhere—bursting at the seams with fifty to seventy-five people inside and out—that they did all the kind things people do when they don't know what to do. And she was very appreciative for the words of comfort that everyone offered, but said that words didn't really help.

With her voice shaking, Sami told me she remembers her friends coming over and saying it was like a movie in reference to all the people and the media there interviewing her and Joanne. And she told her friend, "Yeah, yeah, I guess it's like a movie. But it's not." She said it was good that friends stayed with her and took her out of the house a few times.

Sami doesn't remember talking much with Jacob and Lucas during those days. She said they were around one another and of the same solemn mindset, and just hung around mindlessly watching TV—quiet and filled with sadness and fluctuated between hope and hopelessness.

Sami said all the media came in at the same time, and that she accepted the request for interviews as neither Jacob nor Lucas felt up to being a part of that. She believes that since her emotions were shut down, she could speak and be a part of bringing awareness to the situation, and just wanted it all to be done. She remembers some of it but not all of it, and told me, "All of my memories are either gone or all mixed up."

I agreed with her and shared about my own shutting down, numbness, and going on autopilot. I told her a switch flipped and I knew I had a job to do, and that was to find their father, and that I don't remember much of any tears that were shed in Mexico. It was all shut off, and that there are blanks.

I asked her if her feelings could be described as the glass half empty or half full during those five days, and if she believed her dad was alive in the ocean. She said she didn't think he was alive pretty much from the time Lucas first told her as a result of my phone call. She said she remained very realistic and open to things not going the way that we wanted them to go. She said, "Would I want them to go a certain way? Yeah. But wanting doesn't necessarily give you that. But I didn't say that to anyone. This is probably the first time I've said that. I didn't say it because you have to keep hope alive. But I definitely thought he was gone the whole time. A part of me, of course, didn't want to think that dad was gone. If it turned out dad was alive it would've been a win, win for everyone. I'm not a glass half empty person, but I didn't have the emotions to give anything more because they'd already been turned off."

Sami mentioned the vigil on Friday at The Eagle's Nest Lounge. I told her part of it was a fundraiser to fly her, Jacob, and Lucas to be with me, and she agreed with me that it would have been a bad idea. Sami vaguely remembers being at the vigil and seeing me on the screen. Just like at the house, the restaurant was packed with people and she moved outside after a while to get some fresh air. I told her I remember seeing her, Jacob, and Lucas on my end of the video, and that I emphatically told everyone that it was still a search-and-rescue and *not* a search-and-recovery.

I told her I remember texting at night with her, and that she was my line of survival when I laid in bed throughout the night unable to sleep and my phone would chime, and it was her texting, *Hi mom, are you awake? How are you?* I asked her if we ever talked on the phone, and she believes we talked and texted on Saturday night after David the pilot told me her dad *may never be found.*

Neither of us are sure if I actually said those words to her or if I filtered it to protect her, but Sami was crying that night as she could tell my voice was not as hope-filled as the other days. Sami thinks there was one other time we spoke after her dad's body was found.

I told her how grateful I was that she was there for me each night with the texting. That she was my strength as I laid listening to the taunting waves. Sami said that throughout the five days, she let herself feel just a little bit only with me during the texting, and then again when their dad was found.

I shared with her that I felt talking, instead of texting, would have seemed like a luxury or been considered as a happy or special thing to do. I felt like I didn't deserve to have that. And I did not want to cloud my mind and fill it with anything from anybody. I needed to be there present and focused on the mission to find their dad, and that I had nothing else to offer to anyone. We didn't need to text many words as we were just there for one another. And also, because Patti was lying next to me in the bed, I wasn't going to be talking on the phone. So, it was very simple, not a lot of words, and I told her that I found her few words very comforting and peaceful. I told her I wished we would've kept a copy of all the text messages for our own memories.

One of Sami's last memories of that time is of going to church on Sunday morning with Jacob and Lucas before any of us knew their dad's body had been found. I had requested that the three of them go to church when I spoke to Jacob the day before, on Saturday, when David the pilot went up searching. This was not a typical thing they did together, but because of the circumstances and my request, the three of them went to church. Sami remembers it being an unusually solemn morning, believing in her heart that this was the day they were going to find out something more definite about their dad. She remembers driving to church with her brothers and rocking out to Kesha's new song at the time "C'Mon."

"...I don't wanna think about
What's gonna be after this
I wanna just live right now..."

Sami says Kesha's song affects her still to this day and brings her back to that moment in the car on the way to church.

It is then that I realized that Dave, Patti, and I were probably at church in Mexico at the same time that Jacob, Lucas, and Sami were at church back home.

Sami said she remembers being with her grandma and brothers when I called, and how devastating it was to hear the news, but that they had already prepared themselves for the worst.

I told her how awful a feeling it was for me to not only have to tell them the news of their dad, but not being able to be there with them, and to have to say something like that over the phone was devastating beyond words.

Sami said, "I can't imagine the feeling that you had—that it felt awful, because it sounds awful, and I'm sorry you had to feel that."

When I asked how she felt about picking me up at the airport knowing her dad's ashes were with me, she said she didn't know that, and only remembers being heartbreakingly miserable, very much in the survival mode, and that, "Memories are a crap shoot, you don't necessarily remember what really happened."

We discussed the mourning process and about how people don't 'move on' from grief, that we 'move forward' with it. Sami said with a heavy heart, "Yeah, time heals wounds. Isn't that what they say?"

I said, "I'm not too sure about healing, but that pain takes on different feelings and it's just different, not better."

Sami said at first she didn't talk about losing her dad with anyone, because she felt no one would understand, and she didn't want anyone *hearing her out* because it was a weird thing that had happened. She said people may have reached out to her, but she was pretty dismissive at the time, so she could have simply rejected their compassion without realizing it.

Sami shared that it took her about a year before she started feeling anything. She remembers experiencing a tickle in her chest after the first year and that it felt really weird. And she realized it was because she was coming back out of it. She said she has been more open the last couple of years, as compared to being closed during the previous four to five years. Sami is more reflective and feels closer to her dad, and holds him deep inside her heart more than ever before, because she has been finally able to allow herself to feel both the extreme pain and the profound love for him.

As time moved on, she knew other's whose fathers had died and she had been empathic toward them. She said that through her helping others, she herself in turn had received help—that they developed a symbiotic relationship with each other. She said her way of trying to heal was in reaching out to people who lost their father, and thinking she did it because that is what she herself needed, saying, "The kind of love you give is the kind of love you want." She said she simply likes to listen to others in order to open up a line of communication.

Regarding the MCC Survival Camp, Sami said she still wears the boots that her dad bought a few months prior to his death. I told her I still have the letters that she wrote to us from camp. She was happy to hear that and looks forward to reading them.

I told her, "The reason I need to have our story written is because it's the only thing that will give me peace. And if you, Jacob, or Lucas said to me, no don't write it, I would say I have to because for some reason I keep playing it back in my head over, and over, and over again, and for all these years you would think at some point I could just let it go, but I can't. There are so many significant feelings, emotions, and moments that I don't want to forget, and it just has to be put in writing so that I don't forget. I need to know that every memory that rolls around crazy in my mind is in a format, and that I can finally let it go. Not to let go of the memory of your dad, but the chaos that makes me dizzy in my head. Does that make sense?"

Sami said, "Yes, definitely."

I told her the hope and faith and believing in miracles that we had, is what likely led to her dad's body being found, as the odds were against it. Otherwise, we would have been left with always wondering, still to this day, wondering where he was.

I also told her the reason for writing our story is for people to start understanding how dangerous it can be to travel outside the USA, that the protections and emergency assistance we have in our country is likely not available on the same level elsewhere. And how great it is that there are plans for four lifeguard towers on the beach, and people are being saved every day in large part because of what happened to their dad.

I've asked both Jacob and Lucas if they wanted to share their personal tragedy in losing their dad. Both of them have respectfully declined but fully appreciate their dad's story being told. We continue to share our thoughts and feelings with one another, but they are uncomfortable sharing publicly as it is still very painful. I completely understand and respect their decision.

~~~~~*From Mark's Sisters Missy and Donna: August, 2020*~~~~~

Bonnie and I met with Missy and Donna at my house. They both live nearby, and we settled in my living room as they shared a few special stories they keep near and dear to their hearts about growing up with their brother Mark, and the days leading up to his final day of life.

Donna was the first to tell of childhood stories and said in a trembling voice that, "Even though Mark was ten years older than me; we were extremely close. There was just something so special about him. He was my Mark. We always had a special connection. Mark always showed interest in hearing about things happening in my life. He had a way of looking into your soul with his deep-set sparkling blue eyes and beautiful white smile, and that he was just an amazing person. He always loved. He always cared. He always remembered things I'd told him, and he'd bring them up the next time we saw each other even after a couple of months of not seeing one another.

"As a young girl, Mark used to pay me to make his lunches for him to bring to work. And often when he came home exhausted after working a long, hard day outside, he paid me to take off his dirty work boots and stinky socks. And when Mark blew out his knee and had to have surgery, and his several-week recovery bed was a lawn chair in the basement, I'd run home from elementary school to see him, and make him homemade chocolate frosting that he'd eat straight out of the bowl."

Missy chimed in and said, "When we were younger, Monday night was ice cream night in our house, and Mark would be the last one to eat all of his ice cream. While my brothers and Donna and I quickly gobbled down ours, Mark sat stirring his with a mischievous grin on his face making his ice cream soft and smooth, and then say to the rest of us, 'Oh, look at me. I'm the last one,' as he slowly savored each spoonful in front of us."

Missy laughed and recalled the time when the all-boys Catholic high school Mark attended went co-ed with an all-girls high school, that he started ironing his jeans the first week to impress the girls. But by the end of the second week, he stopped ironing them saying, "I don't care about stupid girls. They don't pay attention to me anyway. I'm going back to being me."

Missy and Donna were enjoying the banter and sharing their memories of their brother, and as each one spoke about a certain situation it jogged a different memory for the other. Donna said Mark loved to joke around and remembered that Mark had purchased a used police car, and one time he had her believing that while he was on the hourlong drive back from one of his softball trips, that he put it on autopilot and the car drove him home while he slept.

Missy, who is five years younger than Mark, remembers that same vehicle and it had a spotlight on the driver's side. She said the two of them would drive up and down alleys in Minneapolis spotlighting kids, and then watch them scatter as the two of them busted out laughing. Missy said Mark tried teaching her how to drive, but quickly gave up when she struggled between knowing the difference between the gas pedal and the brake. Missy and Mark's bond grew even stronger after Missy graduated high school when Mark coached Missy's women's broomball team, and she was thrilled to have him as their coach. During those years, she also went to a lot of Mark's softball games and traveled by bus to his tournaments to places like Virginia, and St. Louis, and that she and Mark had fun together playing co-ed softball with longtime friends and other men and women they'd met over the years.

Donna said, "When I was nineteen, Mark lived in a duplex with our brother Matt, and I loved being around both of them. Mark lived in the upper level and paid me to clean his unit. Mark liked to kid around and would plant extra money in various places, the grimiest places, for me to find and keep when I made my way to that area to clean. I thought that was the funniest thing, and in turn I left him notes in those same areas saying, 'Hey Marky, I was here!'"

The three of us laughed and talked about how stashing things around the house was actually a thing in their household, and both Missy and Donna agreed that their dad used to do the same thing. So Mark learned it from his parents who lived through the Great Depression. It was a common thing for many people in that era, and evidently for some still in our era, as likely that's why Mark did what he did in Mexico when he stashed money around the bungalow.

I told Donna that when Mark and I had started dating about the same time that she cleaned his unit, when I saw her notes, I thought it was so beautiful that they had that special bond, and I told her in our gathering that I still have her notes—that Mark and I had kept them tucked safely away in a folder. It warmed her heart to hear that.

Missy recalled moving into the house that Mark and I bought when we got engaged and she lived in the basement apartment, and the many great times all four of us had together.

Missy shared a time at the house when she had just started dating her now husband, Ken. She said Ken came over to fix her car door, but Mark had never met Ken and didn't know Missy was dating anyone. Ken was bent down nearly to the ground working on her car door when Mark came up behind him wondering who the hell he was, and demanded that Ken tell him what he was doing with his sister's car. Missy said Ken turned to look at who owned the deep, threatening voice, and that his eyes started at Mark's feet and slowly traveled higher and higher up Mark's strong 6'5" frame seeing him standing ready for battle, and that Ken nervously responded saying he knew Missy from work and was just fixing her door.

Donna recalled how Mark used to guard his pizza that he meant only for himself. He always ordered a large sausage and pepperoni with extra sauce from Broadway Pizza with their signature thin crust, and then added his own hot peppers. When their brothers were around, Mark would sit hovering over the pizza with his shoulders and arms circling the outside of the box preventing them from taking a piece—except for Donna, Missy, and me—he was fine with us. Although he probably wished we had our own too, but to his brothers he'd stab their hand with a fork and say, "Order your own. I'll pay for it. Just order your own."

Having been brought up in a family of five with three boys and two girls, in that order, and the boys in their teens well over six feet tall; when the food was put on the table it was gone in a flash as the boys strategically positioned themselves at the table vying for their fair share of the meal. He grew up like that. Dive in or lose out, with his brothers, not with his friends or other people.

I told Donna and Missy if Mark would have ever requested his very last meal it would have been a toss-up between Broadway Pizza or chicken and mashed potatoes with the gravy in the middle, and corn. Burnt corn. I told them I still make corn like that today, and that it's not an easy recipe to duplicate to ensure that it burns just the right amount and doesn't burn to a crisp.

We discussed his honesty and integrity, "The man with a moral compass." We all agreed with each other that Mark didn't judge others but simply took them at their word and face value. And if others said something negative about an individual that Mark knew that seemed out of character, Mark would dismiss it and would continue treating that person respectfully in the manner in which he knew them.

Donna shared how pleased Mark was, at age fifty-eight, to be training heavily in preparation for surfing in Sayulita only months after his rehabilitation from knee surgery in 2012, while also dealing with chronic back pain and other aches and pains resulting from sports injuries and hard work as a lineman for nearly forty years. And I agreed that he wholeheartedly dedicated himself to the training and experienced amazing results both physically and psychologically.

Donna told me how much Mark loved me and our children saying, "You were his Nancy. He just wanted his time with his Nancy and prioritized making time with you and the kids."

Regarding my Tuesday night phone call home on that fateful night of February 26, 2013, Missy said she was home with her husband, Ken. Their oldest son Erik lived nearby with his girlfriend, and Alex was in South Korea. Missy received my phone call routed from an international phone number that she didn't recognize. She often received international calls for work, so she answered it, and it was me saying, "Missy, I've lost Mark." She didn't recognize my voice, just like Lucas didn't recognize mine either.

She said she asked me, "Who is this?"

I told her, "It's me, Nancy, I've lost Mark. I've been running the beach and I can't find him."

Missy said, "Wait, what? What do you mean you've lost him? I don't understand."

She said I explained in a hurried story that, "Mark went swimming, and he hasn't come back, and I think he has been swept out to sea."

And she said she told me, "What? Wait. No, no, no. You're on vacation in a small village and that just doesn't happen."

At that point she said I told her, "I need for you to go to the house with Sami and get the boys to the house, and then call Donna and your brothers and tell them."

She said she was shocked and confused and thought, *No, no I don't know what to tell them!* She said she told me, "Ok, I will do whatever you need." And we hung up. In recalling those horrific seconds, she paused, and with a tear choked voice, she said she looked at her husband, Ken, in shock and disbelief, and told him what I said.

Crippled in their movements, she and Ken packed a bag and went to our house, and on the way, she made the heartrending call to Donna, her voice shaking, telling her, "I need you to go to Nancy's house. Something has happened to Mark. There's been an accident. I don't understand, but we have to get to Nancy's."

Donna said when she received Missy's phone call, she was working late from home, and frozen with the news, she quickly packed a bag and went to our house.

Missy said it broke her heart to have to call their brother's Matt and Mike. When she explained to Matt what I told her and to please come to the house, Matt demanded, "What the hell is going on?"

Missy simply told him, "I don't know, we're going to Nancy's and as soon as I know something I'll call. I just know that something bad has happened."

They arrived at our house around 10 pm and sat with our children with all of them only knowing the scant details that Mark had gone missing in the water. Missy and Donna both said everyone sat around that first night on autopilot questioning what might have happened. Restless: pacing, sitting, talking, not talking, with everyone trying to find ways to offset the pain and confusion. Missy shared how distraught she felt for Jacob, Lucas, and Sami, and that Jacob shared with her that night that he always had a feeling that something bad would happen when his mom and dad traveled. That was his worst fear. And now the worst has happened.

Both Missy and Donna recalled how the house remained filled and busy with love and support from family, their friends, the kids' friends, the workout ladies, and others in the community. Waiting, hoping, and praying. They cooked and baked to pass the time while others brought homemade meals and treats. They talked about the burn hole in the countertop from the hookah pipe coal, and that Lucas told them he hoped their dad would just come home and kick his ass. That all he wanted was for his dad to come home and yell at him for letting that happen. They all just wanted Mark home at all costs. The burn hole did not matter anymore.

Missy said during those nights, after the crowd had left for the evening, she did the last cleanup of the kitchen around 11:30 pm, and afterward would go outside to have a cigarette and look up at the stars saying, "Damnit Mark, I hope you see these same stars I'm looking at right now."

She and Donna stayed at the house the entire week. Missy tried falling asleep in the family room, but she was so wound up and anxious saying she couldn't get comfortable or sit still, and that she busied herself with mindless things like cleaning the bathroom with a toothbrush in an attempt to extinguish the anxiety.

In asking them both if they wished they would have joined me in Mexico, Donna said she would have gone in a heartbeat if I would have asked her, but both she and Missy said they knew that since Dave and Patti were with me, that the best place for them was to be home with Jacob, Lucas, and Sami. We all agreed everyone was where they needed to be during that time.

Donna said, "I don't think there was anyone on this planet that could have brought Mark home. You never gave up. You were so loyal and loving. During the vigil at The Eagle's Nest, you were so incredibly strong, and we knew you weren't coming home without him."

I told both of them that I was hopeful in finding Mark until Saturday when David the pilot told us Mark might never be found, and that I wanted to slap him, thinking, *How dare you say that!*

Donna said until I finally called home on the day he was found five days later, that she never lost hope. With her voice quivering, she said, "I knew in my heart that Mark was okay. I never had a doubt that he'd be found. It was just an awful thought that nobody could find him, but he was the strongest man I ever knew, and I believed he was going to be okay. He was kind. He was smart. God wouldn't allow anything bad to happen to him. He was just beginning the next chapter of his life after working so hard for so many years. When your call came in on the fifth day, our world fell apart. He was gone." And she wiped away tears in her shredded facial tissue that she had been clutching since the beginning of our conversation. And we all wept as we continued sharing and listening to one another.

Donna continued, "On a whim, I brought a pan of apple crisp to the house for Mark, Nancy, and the family the night before they left for Sayulita. I consider it a gift from God that I got to see him one last time. Over the years we all saw each other at family gatherings, but otherwise we were all so busy with our own marriages and raising children, and so for me, that whim turned out to be a major blessing."

Over the years of our marriage, Donna made their mom's mouthwatering apple crisp recipe and would bring it to our house. Others could eat the apple crisp, but it was really intended for Mark. She baked other things, but apple crisp was their special thing. Sometimes Mark was the only one home. And on those occasions, after Donna came and left, Mark would hide wrapped slices of the apple crisp dotted around in the freezer as his own stash. But I knew that if Donna had been to the house, there would have been apple crisp somewhere. Yet, another example of his learned stashing habit.

They both admitted everything from the wake and funeral are just a blur for both of them.

I shared with them the times in our life when Mark told me that when he died, he was going to have to play the 'Nancy Card' in order to get to heaven because of my generosity with It Figures. But it was our generosity together. He downplayed his own giving spirit, and I told him I'd be playing the 'Mark Card' to get to heaven.

Missy and Donna expressed how blessed they were to be at the five-year anniversary of Mark's disappearance with the memorial and tribute of the lifeguard tower listing his name. That out of the tragedy and all of the heartache, that many lives have since been saved and will be saved in the future.

We ended our conversation saying despite the tragedy in losing Mark, that we all feel blessed as a family as we continue to move forward together. It did not tear us apart, and we are always keeping Mark alive.

~~~~~*From My Sister Joanne: August 2020*~~~~~

Bonnie came to my house and we settled in the living room ready for Joanne to share her story.

Joanne said she and Mark had a relationship of funny banter. She recalled that when I first started dating Mark, she had lived in Grand Forks, ND, and that I had asked her to come to Minneapolis so she could meet him. Joanne was hesitant because she had recently had a wisdom tooth pulled and her cheek was swollen. I'd told her not to worry as I'd already told Mark her cheek was puffy and not to make fun of her, and that he agreed he would be nice about it.

Joanne said, "We walked into the bar to meet Mark who was there with his buddies, and Mark stood up to greet me and the first thing he did was puff out his right cheek with his tongue, and said in a garbled voice as if he had a mouth full of cotton, 'Hi nice to meet you.' From that moment on it was always our thing. From time to time throughout the years Mark would do the cheek thing to me. Mark knew how close you and I were and always stood up for me. He had my back. I'd struggled through years of addiction, but Mark never judged me as to what was going on my life. He always just hoped I would get better one day. Mark and I had a good relationship. If I needed a roof over my head, he allowed me to stay with you two and your children, and even a couple of times with me and my children."

And I agree. Mark and Joanne had a warm relationship, and together we were there to support her along the way. Joanne moved in and out of our house over the years of her addiction and she and her son, Aaron, have been living with me since my mom died in 2018. I am so very proud of Joanne as she is now celebrating over seven years of sobriety. It is a godsend having Joanne and Aaron living with me. We have always been close, and growing up we could read each other's minds and finish each other's sentences. She and her ex-husband, Brian, have been through thick and thin together over the years and though he lives in his own house, they're in a strong loving relationship with each other.

At the time Mark died, however, Joanne was living nearby with my mom and that's where she was when I called home the night Mark disappeared. Joanne said she answered her phone and that I told her in a shaky voice, "Joanne, I've lost Mark!"

Joanne said she nervously chuckled, "What do you mean you've lost Mark?"

I told her, "He's gone. I've lost Mark and you need to get to my house right now. The kids are going to be there, and you need to tell them he's gone."

Joanne said her body went numb and her head started swirling thinking *what the hell is going on here? This isn't real!* And she asked me, "Are you joking around?"

I said, "No, I'm not joking. You need to get to the house now and be there with the kids."

Joanne said with her head in a fog she quickly packed some things for her and our mom, who was also completely flustered with the news, and they drove to our house. When they got to the house, Jacob, Lucas, and Sami were home and knew from my call to Lucas that their dad had gone missing. It was just Joanne, our mom and the kids at the time. I told her the only call I remember, as I've told the others who said I called them, that I only remember speaking to Lucas. Joanne said I had told her she was the first person I called, and that people just started coming to the house with everyone's minds in a state of confusion wondering, *what the hell is going on,* while waiting for more calls from me, and that the children were completely distraught.

Joanne remembers Dave and Patti walking through the door that night and Dave saying, "We're going to Sayulita. We've got a flight for tomorrow morning." She wanted to go with them, but Dave told her no, that she needed to stay and manage the house.

Joanne said, "A lot of people continuously came and went bringing food, well wishes and prayers. There were many phone calls with people asking what they could do, and a lot of downtime with a few of us sitting around the table, and many others in the house waiting. Kim was the main point of communication for finding out about the news stories, and was one of the key people at the house, along with Missy and Donna, with other people coming and going. It was just one big waiting game. Waiting for a phone call from you. Just waiting for news of any kind. We watched the news reports, but I hadn't talked to you since you called me the night Mark disappeared. I was at the house trying to maintain everything and take care of the kids because they were like ghosts floating around the house. There—but not there. Not knowing what to say to anyone. Not wanting to talk to anyone. They were in their own little worlds. People used different coping mechanisms to try to numb the pain. Some of it included shutting down, anger, food, and alcohol. I was only six months sober and around alcohol. It was *hell* for me. I had to tell myself, *No! No! No!* I felt I had strength from Mark calling to me saying, *Joanne you can do this.* There's no other logical reason I stayed sober at that time."

I told Joanne that was another big hurdle she had to overcome during that time. We both agreed that it would have been the easiest excuse in the world for her to start drinking again. And I said to her, "It's as if Mark handed you strength and accountability with Mark whispering, *Joanne, this is your time to shine.*

Joanne agreed, "Yes, my time for you, with Mark telling me, *Nancy needs you here and sober to take control of things.* I get goose bumps thinking about it because I felt a distinct sensation come over me, and thought, *I can't let Nancy down this time. I've let her down all these years.*

I can't do it again. I developed strength. It was just a quick moment that this happened as I stood next to the coffee maker, and beside that sat a large bottle of vodka which was my weakness. I looked at it and said to myself, *I can do this. And I'm gonna do this.* And from that moment on, with only six months of sobriety, it didn't bother me not to drink and be around others who were. I'd spent thirty years as an addict and relapsed many times along the way, but I overcame it with a sudden inexplicable strength from within. I could easily have drunk with no one noticing unless I'd gotten so wrecked that it was obvious. Yet, I did not take a sip. I wouldn't go there. And I did it for the entire five days before we received news that Mark had died, and I've been sober ever since. I truly believe the strength came from Mark coming to me."

I said to her, "If you would've relapsed again in mourning Mark's disappearance because of your aggressive relapses, that it likely would've killed you, and that this tragedy in losing Mark was the ultimate test in your sobriety."

"Yes, it was the ultimate test," Joanne replied, "there's no reason why I stayed sober. It was as if Mark was standing over me encouraging me with the inner strength he himself possessed. And so, I did what I had to do to keep the house organized along with Missy and Donna and the others, and be there for Jacob, Lucas, and Sami."

Joanne said she went home every night to stay with our mom, and that after getting mom settled each morning at her home in the beginning stages of Alzheimer's, she returned to our house for the remainder of the day. Mom had believed that everything was going to be okay with Mark no matter what.

Joanne said, "The days went on and on and when we found out about the vigil that would be happening on Friday night, I was so excited to finally see your face, along with Dave and Patti, and the environment you were in. I was happy to know everyone was still hopeful, and to hear your words of it being a search-and-rescue and not a search-and-recovery with David the pilot going in the air the next day. After the vigil, many people came back to the house and waited some more. And on Saturday, the house filled with even more people waiting for news of the search-and-rescue. Again, just a big waiting game."

Joanne said she is not sure how she found out that Mark had not been found on Saturday, that it could have been Sami or Kim, and that I said I was not coming home until Mark was found.

I told her I talked to Sami that night and maybe that's how word got out. I told her my mind shut down even more after the pilot said Mark may never be found, and that I prayed the novena prayer during the night, and Mark came to me just before dawn saying they know the location.

Joanne said, "On Sunday, the house became packed again after you called me saying you had news and to get the kids and mom together at the house. People asked me what I knew, and I told them I don't know anything, I'm waiting for information. It was just crazy around the house. Everything a blur. When the kids and mom went into the room to receive your phone call, everyone in the house just looked around at each other until mom came out of the bedroom and sadly told us—Mark is gone—he drowned in the ocean. Then, there was a big whoosh of release in tension when the unknown became known. It was done. We all knew Mark was gone, and everyone began consoling one another throughout the day as more food came in and then people slowly left the house. Over the next couple of days, we organized and cleaned the house preparing for your return. It was a form of relief that Mark was found—but not really."

I told Joanne I understood about feeling relief and that is what I felt when the fireman told me they found his body.

Joanne said, "I was the only one in the house when you and the kids returned from the airport, as I wanted to be there to comfort you, and I stood in the doorway wanting to grab you and hug you, but you looked straight through me like I wasn't there, and it hurt at the time. Though I didn't blame you, it did hurt."

I told her I didn't remember that and that I didn't mean to hurt her. Joanne said the kids and I went straight into the back room together, and that she went home and came back the next morning. I told her that I don't remember her standing there, and that maybe since we're so close and know each other so well that she'd understand I just needed to be with my children—and that it wasn't a conscious effort on my part. I didn't want to give my attention to anyone but them. I explained to her that it's crazy how I blacked out so many things during those several days. I told her I was glad for her story, and the story of others, to fill in the blanks. We discussed how so much of it was a blur for so many people. Upon hearing horrific news your mind and body go into shut down and survival mode at the same time. That it's odd as to what is so vivid and what becomes fuzzy and even forgotten.

We discussed the fact that when Sami heard from Lucas of my phone call home that she immediately didn't think Mark was alive, and that she 'put on' to others the hope they had, but that she herself didn't have the same hope.

Joanne shared that she didn't carry that hope either and felt Mark was gone right away. She said, "I never believed he was alive probably because when he came to me and passed along his strength to me, I knew he was gone and watching over me the entire time. I felt his presence."

I shared with Joanne that I had many visits with Mark for up to six months after he died, and in one of them she and I were out in the boonies somewhere in the desert driving on a dusty dirt road, and I was upset with her terrible driving. We pulled up to a bar and sat down in the couch area and Mark was next to me. I knew he was dead, yet he was talking to me, but I didn't want to look at him too closely because I thought he would go away. I asked other people if they could see him, and they said yes. And I said, *No, you don't understand, he is dead.*

Mark said, *What are you talking about?*

Mark, you drowned. I said.

And he was very confused by it all asking, *How can I be here with you if I'm gone?*

I don't pretend to know the ins and outs of the afterlife and the extent to which our deceased loved ones communicate with us and what they understand, however, I do believe it is real.

And some may question that visits do occur. All I know is it happened, and I know there's much research that exists in the scientific realm about what may happen to our spirit's consciousness after our heart stops beating, and that myriads of people around the world have experienced visits from their deceased loved ones.

I'm a dreamer and know the difference between a dream and a visit. And the first visit I ever had was with my mother-in-law. For me, the distinction between a dream and a visit is that when I'm experiencing a visit, I know I'm sleeping, and I'm having a conversation. I'm very aware that I'm sleeping, and that the other person should not be talking to me. However, in a dream people don't interact with me like that.

I had about six other visits with Mark during the next few months, and one time was especially memorable. We were on a beautiful, peaceful beach somewhere at a non-descript location. I absolutely knew, while I was sleeping, that Mark was gone, and it was a fantastic feeling of being fulfilled having spent time with him. Again, I didn't look straight at him fearing that he would disappear, and I told him I wish I could have been a better wife as I thought about the financial disappointments that I had caused with the club, and felt guilty overextending on things like the many large events we had at our house and elsewhere. And Mark said, *No, you were everything I needed and wanted.* And said he thought the club was necessary and important for me and so many people.

Both Joanne and I acknowledged the reality of visits with people who have died. We both have had visits with our dad and mom, and Joanne with our grandma, and I've had a couple of visits with Mark's deceased mother.

Joanne then reminded me about a phone call she had received while I was in Mexico from a woman who had been a member of It Figures. She is a local medium and told Joanne that I needed to know that it happened in an instant, that Mark didn't feel any pain. That the wave that came down hit him like cement, and he didn't suffer. Joanne had told me that on the day after I returned home from Mexico, and I simply took it at face value, and never called the woman asking for more information. While I believe the gifts of mediums are real, I'm not one who searches for a deeper meaning to life in that manner. I can only testify to the visits I've had with Mark, our mom and dad, and Mark's mom.

~~~~~*From Kim and Joe: August 2020*~~~~~

My friend Kim and her husband, Joe, came to my house to share their story with Bonnie and me, and we settled in my living room. They talked about our times together as a foursome and when they first found out Mark was missing.

Kim reminisced saying, "When you're a married couple, you always want another couple that you can hang out with, and even feel free to argue in front of each other. The four of us traveled to Mexico and Las Vegas and spent Valentine's dinners together. We were together for many life events including deaths. In fact, I was there when Mark's dad died. It just happened that my mom was in the same nursing home as his dad, and I was visiting my mom when Mark and Nancy's family were at the nursing home when Mark's dad passed away. One thing I miss since Mark has been gone is 'us.' The four of us. It was always the four us. Mark was frugal, so often our time together meant just hanging out at Mark and Nancy's house. Sometimes Nancy and I would hang out and the guys would go watch golf in the other room."

When they heard about Mark's disappearance, Kim said, "Joe and I were at home eating dinner and a friend called me asking if it was true that Mark was missing. I had no idea what she was talking about. She just told me all she heard was that Mark went missing, and I turned to Joe telling him Mark went missing."

Joe recalled saying to Kim, "What? Whaddya mean he's missing? Did he walk off into the sunset on the beach or something? And Kim told me her friend said that Mark was swimming and got swept away by a wave. I froze, and my only response was, holy shit."

Neither Kim nor Joe remembers anything else from that night except spending the remaining hours in shock.

Kim and Joe said they went to the house the next day, and like the others, commented about the large gathering of people at our house sitting and standing around in disbelief.

Joe said he sat at a table with Mark's brothers, Matt and Mike, and said to them, "There is no way that Mark drowned. He is a strong swimmer, and we had body surfed and swam together in the ocean numerous times over the years. Something happened where he got swept out, but he has to be out there alive. And until they find him or find a body, I'm not going to believe he's gone, and that Mike and Matt agreed with me."

But then later that morning, Joe said he searched satellite data of the waves on the day Mark went missing and followed the current map from Puerto Vallarta up the coastline to Sayulita, and that he said to himself, *Oh my god,* that even though he knew it was a surfing village, there was white water everywhere and he could see the turbulence. He shared what he found with Mark's brothers, and the three of them believed Mark might not have survived it after all, but that they did not share their beliefs with others.

I interjected telling them that we all had hope in Sayulita. That even five days into the search David the rescue and recovery pilot said, 'no body' was better than 'a body,' and that there was a chance Mark could be alive stranded on an island somewhere or hanging onto debris.

We discussed how distraught Kim's niece had been after Kim told her about Mark disappearing the night before, just minutes before her niece went into a staff meeting at KSTP-TV, and that throughout the meeting her head was in a fog, and then afterward one of the reporters pulled her aside asking what was wrong. At that time, her niece didn't know if she had permission to divulge the news and presented a 'what if I know' scenario about a Minnesota husband and father who went missing in Mexico on vacation. The reporter told her it was important news, and if publicizing the situation could help, it was vital to get the news out. And KSTP-TV became the first local station to air the story on Wednesday; interviewing me over the phone with a photo of Mark and me inset on the screen.

Kim said everyone at the house had gathered around the television in worried, heartrending anticipation of the news report. Kim also commented about the plentiful food piled high, how terribly difficult it was for Jacob, Lucas, and Sami; that Missy, Donna, and Joanne were like fixtures at the house, and how amazingly strong Joanne had been staying sober through it all.

Joe said he had a golf vacation planned to Florida with a bunch of guys that he wanted to cancel, but Kim told him no, that Mark would have wanted him to go. Hesitantly, Joe went knowing there was nothing he could do by either staying home or going on the trip, and knew that Kim would keep him updated on the developments of the search. Joe remembers standing over every putt saying to himself, *Come on Mark, help me put this in the cup.*

Kim said she knew I was not going to come home without Mark, either alive or dead, and that she and Joe had already decided they would come and spend time with me, either together or trade time between themselves, until he was found.

Kim commented how strong I was to have spoken at the wake and the funeral the next day. But I told her I had to address people to tell them what happened to Mark, and to show my gratitude for their outpouring of love and support.

Kim said their daughter, Maddie, was only nine years old when Mark died and Maddie asked her, "I don't understand mom, why did it happen? Mark was so big and strong; I just don't get why he died." Kim said she told her that the ocean took him away, and we always have to look at the ocean and pray and think of Mark and grandma, because Kim's mom had died before Mark, and that her mom's wishes were to have her ashes spread over the ocean in the area where they vacationed in Florida.

Joe said Maddie wouldn't let him go into the ocean when on vacation in Florida for two years after Mark's death, even though the water at the location where they went to the ocean had little to no wake.

Kim agreed with Joe saying Maddie wouldn't let Joe go in the water, pleading with him, *Dad, you're not going in the ocean. You're going to drown just like Mark!*

However, Kim said, "Now that Maddie is older, she now drags Joe into the ocean."

I told them I never knew that and shared with them a time when Maddie and I went for a walk in a nearby park six years after Mark had died. We walked over a stream on a wooden bridge and Maddie said to me, "I smell Uncle Mark."

He was her godfather, not her uncle, but that's how she referred to him. I told them I was taken aback and looked at Maddie, then at the bridge, and saw that it was coated heavily with creosote, and asked her if she knew *why* it smelled like Uncle Mark. I explained to Joe and Kim that I told Maddie that Mark smelled like creosote from the power poles. It was almost like his aftershave. It didn't matter if he took a shower and scrubbed down, it was in the fiber of his clothing, boots, on his skin, and inside his car. He smelled like a lineman. I told them I can't smell a power pole without smelling Mark.

We discussed going to Sayulita for the first-year anniversary of Mark's death and staying in Nuevo Vallarta while visiting Sayulita just for the day. Kim was with us and reminded me that I wasn't on board with anyone swimming in Sayulita, but was okay with swimming in Nuevo Vallarta as the waters are far calmer there. Kim recalled returning to Nuevo Vallarta later that day, and that at sunset I dove furiously into the waves a couple of times. She said it looked like I was angry at the waves. Kim said everyone in our party witnessed me diving forcefully into the waves and that many were surprised I went into the water at all. And Kim said she told them, "If that's how Nancy feels in order to connect with Mark, then that's how she feels."

That is the only time I went into the ocean on that trip, and my brother Dave took a silhouetted photo of me walking into the ocean toward the sunset that I keep close to my heart; not only for the memory of me entering the same ocean about twenty nautical miles south of the waters that took *my* Mark from me one year earlier at that same time of day, but because Kim had given me a very similar silhouetted photo, with a near identical sunset, that she had taken of both Mark and me in Puerto Vallarta on one of our previous couple's vacations together. I keep both photos next to each other on my bedroom wall.

Mark and me in Puerto Vallarta in 2011

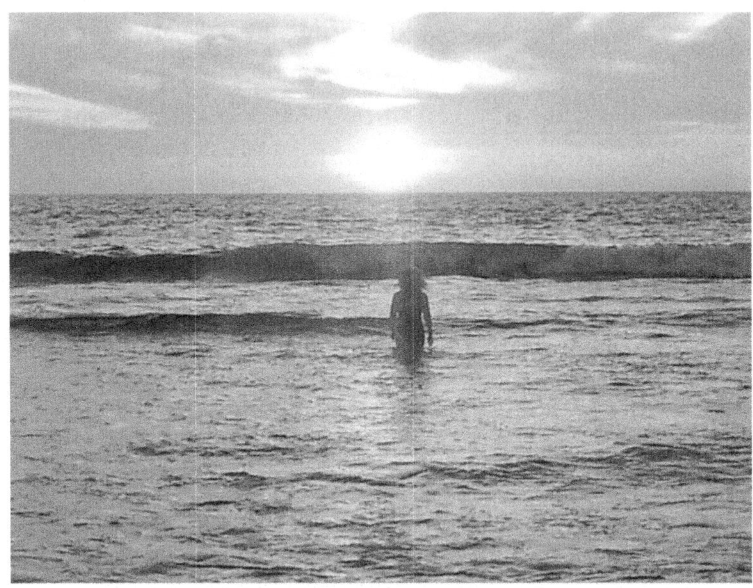

Me walking into the same Puerto Vallarta waters in 2018.

Joe said in June 2020, seven years after Mark's death, he was working in a new house in the local area, and they had extension cords running throughout the house to a generator because the power was out. The owner of the house said Xcel Energy was expected at any time to repair the outage, and then shortly thereafter an Xcel truck showed up. Joe said he took a break and intentionally went to talk to the Xcel worker to ask him if he knew Mark Stoneberg.

The worker looked at Joe surprised, "Yeah, you mean Stoney? I was just a snot-nosed kid when he taught me the ropes, and I swear to God, there's not a day that goes by that we don't mention his name or say something that Mark used to say, because Stoney always had his little sayings like *what's your point, or what part of no don't you understand?*"

Joe and I discussed how great a role model Mark was to those he trained and an example to fellow linemen as well, and agreed that Mark never turned down overtime. He always answered the phone from Xcel after hours thinking it would mean overtime.

Joe then said, "Nancy, you've asked me to go down there a few times and I've always declined, because I don't want to see the evil place that took Mark. I have no desire to go there." And to this day Joe has not visited anywhere in Mexico since Mark's death. He still visits the ocean, but no longer in Mexico.

I explained to Joe that I understood his feelings, and explained to him why it was important for me to go back there even if no one came with me. I told him it's because of what happened between Mark and me from the time we were on the airplane until Tuesday night when he disappeared—that our time together was like never before in our marriage. I shared with him how Mark had woken up pain-free in a rustic village atmosphere, not a fancy resort, and that his face glowed from the moment he got into the shuttle in Puerto Vallarta.

~~~~~From Liz of Liz and Kirk: September 2020~~~~~

Liz came to my house to share her story with Bonnie and me and we settled at the kitchen island. We met with her on 9/9/20, and she commented that she had first met Mark nine years ago almost to the day on 9/10/11.

Liz and I reminisced about the small intimate New Year's party at our house just a few weeks before our trip to Sayulita playing stupid little games, and having contests in our basement gym. I told her how unique and special it really was to share that time with Mark before he died.

We laughed about the suitcase filled with food with me not declaring it, and then Kirk urging me to place it next to Old Sac to bring through customs as he would do better in jail than I would.

Liz and I recalled the selfie on the shuttle bus which was the first selfie I'd ever taken, and how super happy we all were. Liz remembered us getting dropped off at the trailer park and trudging along the sand dragging suitcases to the bungalow, and Mark seeing the bananas in the trees yelling, "Nancy Elizabeth! Nancy Elizabeth! There's bananas in that tree!"

I told her again how enthralled Mark had been with every aspect of being there in that newfound slice of paradise.

Liz reminisced about the beautiful horse dancing and the reaction from the waitress at the restaurant when she realized that it was the two tall, strong men who ordered the fruity slushy ones, and ours were the regular one's on the rocks.

Liz talked about how wild, loud, and continuous the waves were that Tuesday morning as she and I sat on the beach with the guys gone surfing. She agreed the ocean was unlike any other day on our trip, and that she sent a video to her daughters because it was so unusual. I told Liz that I give her credit for helping to save the life of the man lying in the water that day because he was out of my line of sight, and that if she didn't see *something* in the water, he likely would have drowned as he was motionless and face down in the water when I got to him, and no one else had gone to his rescue.

Liz recalled commenting to Mark about his unusually sparkling eyes and white teeth as we sat in their loft area prior to heading down the beach with the guys for one more session of body surfing, before going to dinner at the swing chair restaurant.

She said on Saturday night, the night before Mark's body was found, that she had begged and pleaded with God saying we need to find Mark. We *cannot* leave here without him.

Liz spoke about the many people from the village who came to the beach memorial and the G-O-D dog that sat next to me. She asked if I remembered a surfer dude who came and knelt before me, bawling, with his head down, holding my hand and saying he was so sorry. I told her I don't remember that. She said she and Kirk thought that because the guy was so broken up, that likely he was one of the paddle boarders with FFCB looking for Mark the night he went missing, and on the other days as well.

Liz and I talked about how Mark's story, our journey, has morphed into something more spiritual after thinking about everything that happened toward the end of Mark's life leading up to his death. Liz said Kirk has talked about the look in Mark's eyes in a photo taken when he, Mark, and others were in Pebble Beach together in 2012. That Mark's eyes were so at peace knowing he was nearing retirement with a sense of accomplishment in his career and finances, and how well he had taken care of his family. I have a copy of that photo, and agree that even though Mark truly enjoyed life during his fifty-eight years of life on this earth, he looked forward to enjoying it more freely on his own time schedule.

Kirk and Liz have been back to Sayulita twice since 2013, and Kirk has taken time to be alone where Mark disappeared. He has been back to the north end of the beach, with the gigantic boulders where people build rock memorials, to build a new one like he and Liz first made for Mark. Kirk gave me a copy of a photo he took of the memorial he made with a picture of Mark next to it, and I treasure it deeply. The picture is of Mark sitting in an extra, extra, large folding camp chair designed for two people, but with Mark's big, strong stature—the chair looks like it was made just for him.

I've asked Kirk if he wanted to share about his personal tragedy in losing his dear friend, Mark, but he has respectfully declined as he does not feel comfortable sharing publicly about his loss. I completely understand and respect his decision.

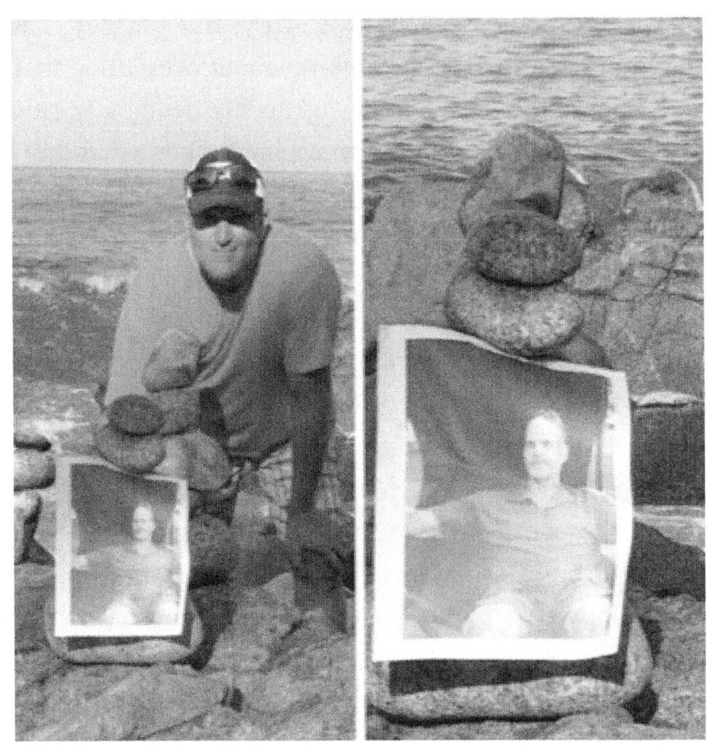

Kirk at Mark's Rock Memorial in Sayulita

~~~~*Delta Pilot, Rob Reed—December 2020*~~~~

Over the years I had wanted to connect with the Delta pilot from my church who flew me home from Sayulita with me carrying Mark's ashes in my suitcase, but the opportunity never presented itself. I'd always wondered how he knew who I was and how he turned out to be our pilot that day. I hadn't seen him in a few years, and I recently asked our church administrator if she knew how to contact him. She said he was no longer of member of our parish, but she had his phone number and gave it to me.

I called Rob and he was very receptive to my phone call and asking him questions. He reminded me that he and I did talk one time after Mark's death at a church function shortly after Mark's funeral. He said he was in

Puerto Vallarta and was going to be flying back to Minneapolis on that Tuesday, and that his wife had heard about Mark's death at church that morning. Rob said his wife asked Father Pederson for more details, and he told her I was flying home that same day, so his wife texted him explaining the situation and informed him I was flying back that same day also.

Rob explained that when he got to the airport, he checked the list and saw my name. He said he didn't know what I looked like, but that his wife explained to him that I'd taught their child for First Communion and described me as short with red curly hair, and that's how he found me in the terminal. He told me that he described what I looked like to the flight attendants, explained what had happened to Mark, and asked them to make me as comfortable as possible. He said he didn't ask them to put me in first class, that they did that on their own when they saw there was an empty seat.

Rob said he had looked for Mark's casket in the special cargo area on the airplane reserved exclusively for the deceased, but he couldn't find it. I told him Mark's ashes had been in my carry-on bag. He said the experience of tragically losing a spouse in and of itself would have been traumatic for anyone, but especially if you hadn't intended for a cremation and then to be holding the ashes in a carry-on bag. And he went on to share that twenty-two years prior, his first wife had died, and though our losses were different, he remembers the pain of being a young widower and could feel the pain of my loss.

Rob's kindness once again overwhelmed me, and I thank him for helping to fill in another missing piece of the mosaic in our lives before Mark's disappearance, and in the troubling, horrible days that followed.

I am grateful to Sami, Dave and Patti, Missy and Donna, Joanne, Kim and Joe, Liz, and Rob for sharing their thoughts and feelings. Each conversation provided further healing for me as each one of them helped to fill in missing pieces, and it offered a certain sense of healing for each person as well, because none of us had previously shared with one another the depths of our experiences. While I'd often told others of the chaos in Mexico, I told the stories almost from a superficial level, telling the facts of scenes rolling around in my head, but not letting others into the far-reaching depths of my feelings. Maybe that was about self-preservation. Yes, we share stories about Mark all the time, and people remember and live within their own deep feelings, and the deeper feelings have sometimes surfaced and have been shared, but only in fragments if they were shared at all. However, in each session, any suppressed emotions that may have existed with anyone, were allowed the opportunity to arise and flow freely.

I don't remember anything more after that call to Lucas that first evening when in actuality I'd called, Joanne, my brother Dave, Missy, and Kim. That's the bizarre thing about all of this. The fact that your brain can shut things out like that, is scary. Because I can remember other things 'to a T.' But that's really one of the things that has haunted me over and over still today—not remembering some details. So again, I'm grateful for everyone who has helped fill in the blanks and refine the blur.

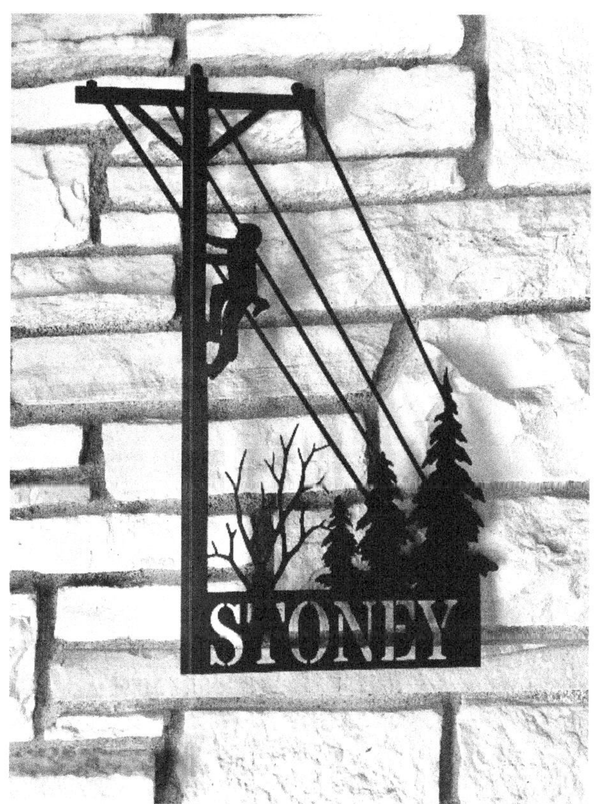

I had 3 of these made for my children.

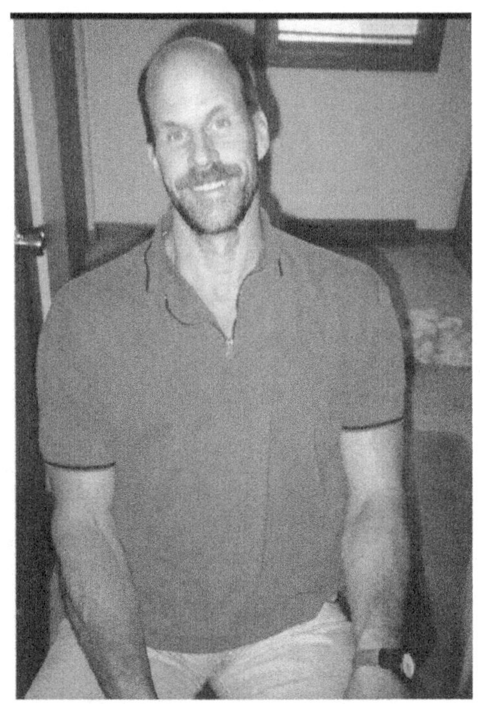

Mark

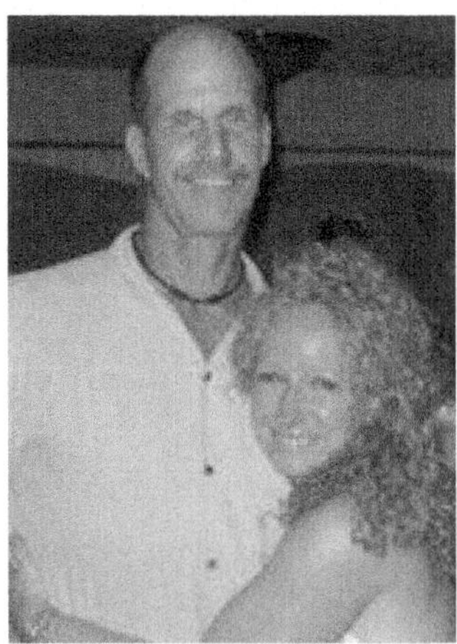

A favorite photo of Mark and me

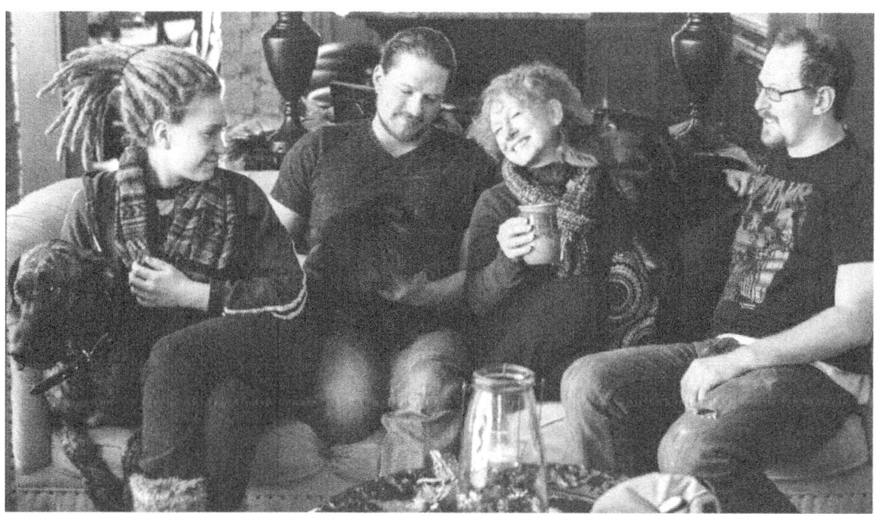

Dog Dolce, Sami, Jacob, Dog Buffy, Me, Dog Chaser, and Lucas

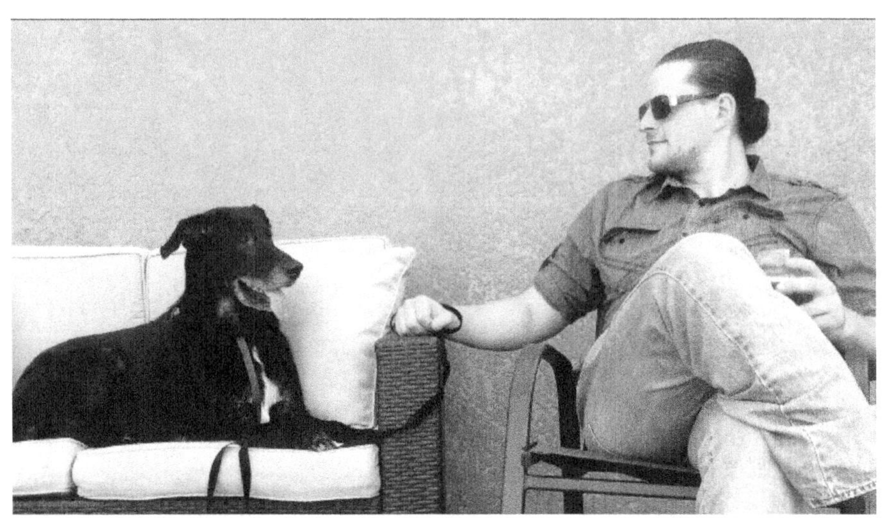

Chaser and Jacob

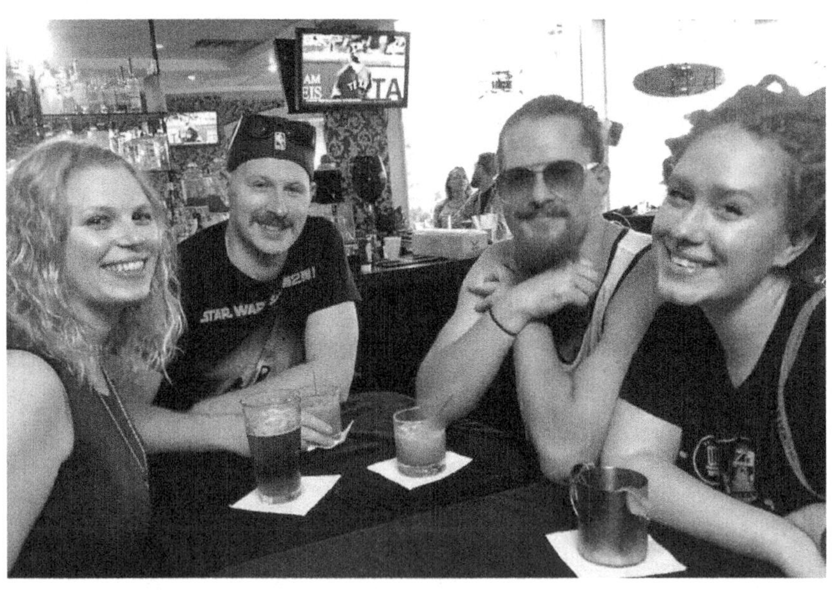

Kati, Lucas, Jacob, and Sami

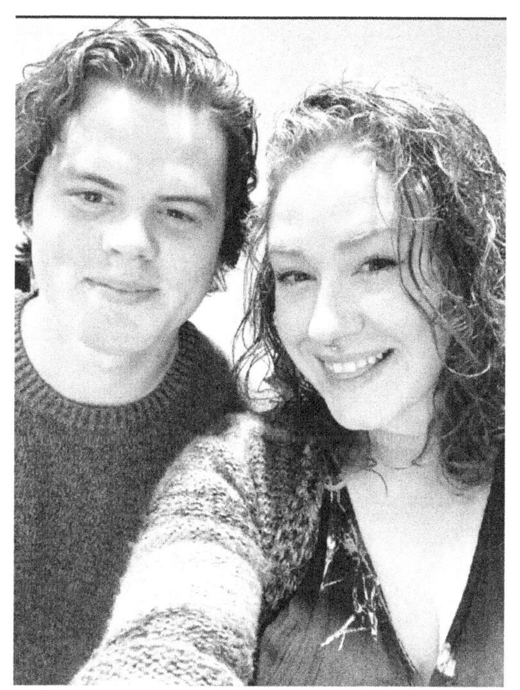

Aaron and Sami

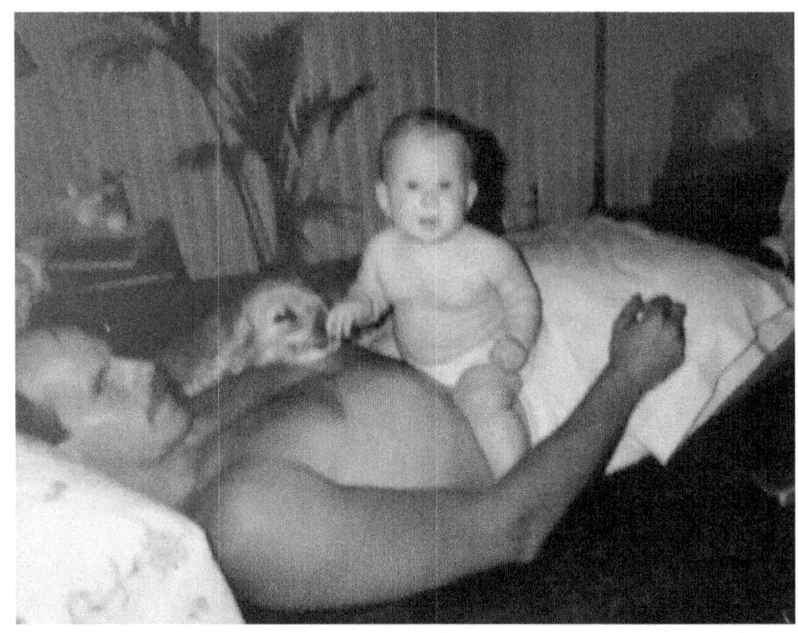

Mark and Jacob

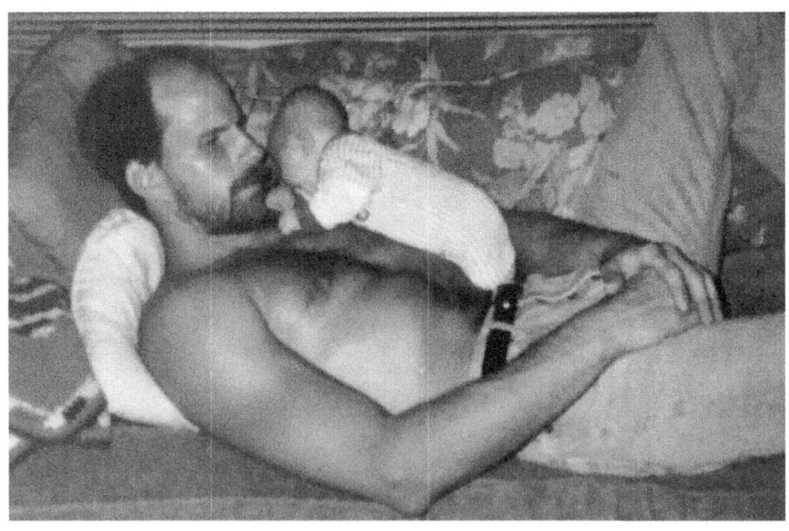

Mark and Lucas

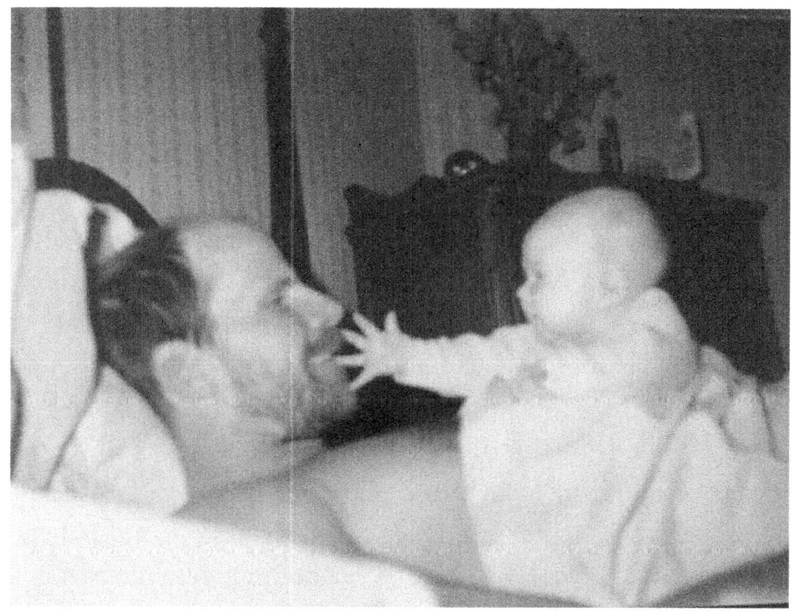

Mark and Sami

NANCY'S POSTSCRIPT

This journey of mine has never been about the one. It has been about the many. The many people who have supported me and my family over these last several years. While it may be possible to list everyone along the way, I fear in doing so I might mistakenly leave out just one person due to a simple oversight or lapse in memory, so I have chosen to thank everyone in the following manner:

Family, my friends, Mark's friends, It Figures community of women, Birdtown friends, Bootcamp/Coffee Group, local TV and newspapers, Sacred Heart Church community, Robbinsdale business and government communities, Mark's coworkers, David the search pilot, Rob Reed the Delta Pilot, Dan Delmore, the consulate representative, Janice along with the other Pro Sayulita volunteers, and the FFCB for their life saving mission in Sayulita.

The words, "Thank you," cannot possibly come close to the gratitude and appreciation I feel towards Bonnie. We have been friends since our children were young but had not seen each other for a few years. She appeared out of nowhere to help me move beyond the dizzying thoughts that had me bound. Her strength, kindness, compassion, and patience over the past two years of writing have been nothing less than heroic. She certainly is nothing less than another one of those blessed miracles brought to me by the grace of God! Her profound and talented gift of writing has been astounding. I am forever grateful for her dedication during this journey of healing. The past two years with Bonnie have been a beautiful gift through meeting in person, and remotely by phone with recorded sessions, to co-create the story in losing *our* Mark, and I'm looking forward to many more years of time together!

I'm fortunate to say that as a result of working through this story and getting both the good and tragic events of those days in Sayulita in writing, that it has been therapeutic. With that said, I still feel sick to my stomach when thoughts come to mind when I felt 100% sure that Mark remained alive in the water or beached somewhere, and the hopelessness he would've felt every night at sunset knowing he'd be spending another night in the cold dark blackness of the ocean. I could not get my head around it then and I still cannot to this day. The deep-rooted wounds will always remain. And it is only by God's grace that I survived without going mad in the process.

I will always and forever remember those events and feel both the joy of our time together and the pain of losing Mark, but not having to force my mind to remember so that I don't forget, is freeing.

It has been nine years since Mark's passing and seven years since my fiftieth birthday pledge to travel the USA and other countries by the age of sixty-five, and I'm still on track for that goal having visited eight states and six countries— though it slowed down due to COVID-19.

Jacob lives near me. Lucas and his fiancé, Kati, live nearby as well. Sami and her boyfriend, Aaron, live in Oregon, and Joanne and her son, Aaron, live in the upstairs apartment of my home. I'm now in a healthy and loving relationship with Jeff Kuba who I was blessed to meet five years after Mark's passing.

BONNIE'S POSTSCRIPT

I have been richly blessed in my longtime friendship with Nancy, and am grateful and honored to have been part of helping her work through her and her family's tragic journey in losing Mark. Though Nancy didn't physically write the story, she and I worked it and re-worked it every step of the way together, similar to a director, co-producer, and writer relationship with a wonderful synergy between the two of us.

Nancy is an articulate speaker and vivid storyteller. I had been brought to tears many times during our live meetings and remote recording sessions listening to Nancy describe the horrific events in losing Mark, and again when writing about those same events while attempting to capture the emotional and physical depths of her soul during that time. I remain inspired by Nancy's courage in the midst of this unimaginable tragedy.

It has been a sacred endeavor for me. I pressed myself to try to feel the hell that she endured throughout the several nights and days, and the similar hell that Jacob, Lucas, and Sami endured back home. I pushed myself to try to capture the misery that Kirk and Liz, and Dave and Patti endured in Mexico, and the other family members and friends suffering back home. In attempting to drive myself emotionally into their struggles, my hope is that I did justice to everyone in the process.

I am thankful that this writing has allowed Nancy to heal even though the indelible scars of her tragedy remain.

On a final note, when Joe, of Kim and Joe, shared his story about his encounter with an Xcel lineman in June 2020, my heart melted because I too came across an Xcel lineman in September 2020 doing repairs at our neighbor's house, and asked him if he knew Mark Stoneberg. He said he had been at Xcel for ten years and trained under Mark, and that he was a great guy—a legend—and that they still talk about him today.

ACKNOWLEDGEMENTS

We offer a special thanks to:

Mark's sister, Missy, for reading our initial draft and offering priceless feedback regarding our family's heartbreaking reality in losing our Mark.

Bonnie's husband, Bob, for reading our initial draft and offering insightful observations.

Lynda Tysdal, who offered vital information about the publishing process.

Susan Gallagher, for reading the manuscript, offering discernment with the flow, and a special heartfelt reaction to our story.

Bonnie's brother, Joe Egan (joeegan.com), for also reading the manuscript and offering invaluable feedback, as well as connecting us to our editor, Mandi.

Mandi Spaid, our editor, who provided us with her amazing expertise with editing, publishing, and marketing. She can be found at WritersBlockInc.com under her pen name.

Tom Butler, who benevolently managed the CaringBridge posts, and developed our website: www.stoneybook.com.

Kim Dehn, who was my support, and connection with the media and helped with the CaringBridge posts.

Janice Parker, along with Pro Sayulita and FFCB, who continue in their devotion to keep the beaches in Sayulita safe, and for the commemorative first lifeguard tower bearing Mark's name.

A portion of the proceeds from the sale of *Stoney* will go to Pro Sayulita for their lifesaving efforts.

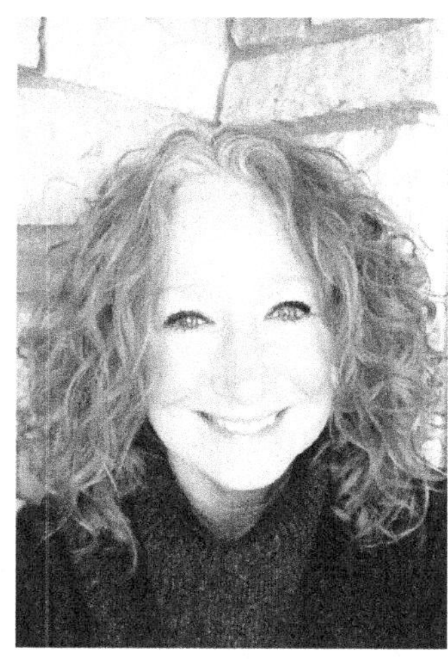

Nancy Stoneberg is a gifted professional speaker and inspirational presenter. She has served as a planning commissioner for the City of Robbinsdale, co-owned the women's fitness club, It Figures in Robbinsdale, and has appeared numerous times on KSTP-TV's, *Twin City's Live* as their 'fitness guru.' Nancy is most content living "in the action." With her kindhearted and free-spirited personality she easily draws people together, and can be found most often with family and friends gathering inside her warm and welcoming kitchen, and outside in her lush garden paradise. You may visit her via the web:

Website: https://www.stoneybook.com

Website: https://nancystoneberg.com

Facebook: https://www.facebook.com/nancy.stoneberg

Instagram: https://www.instagram.com/nstoneberg/

YouTube:
https://www.youtube.com/channel/UCR2OGKI33Djd6MRCFyVJc8g

Linkedin: https://www.linkedin.com/in/nancy-stoneberg-01412425

Twitter: https://twitter.com/thestonefitness?lang=en

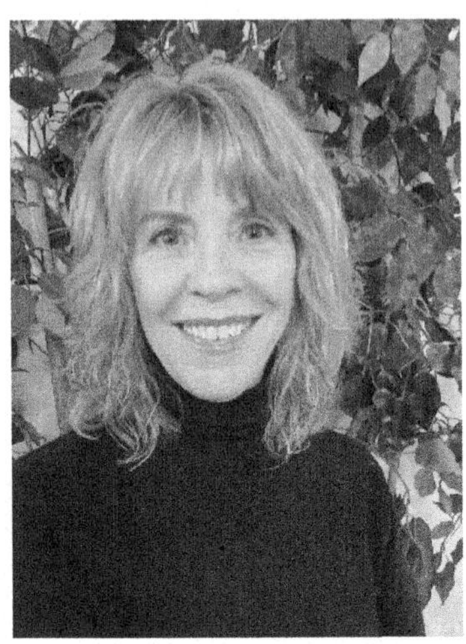

Bonnie's writing collection also includes a children's rhyming earth science picture book manuscript, mature readers fiction manuscript in development, and collection of poetry and song lyrics. Throughout her careers in business and education, she has created training manuals and curriculum for adult English language learners, and she is a gifted trainer and presenter.

When she is not writing in her favorite alcove, Bonnie works full-time and spends much time with her family and delving into her other passions of reading, genealogy research, music, and transforming her backyard into a tranquil wonderland.

Aside from social media, Bonnie is well connected in the community and has an expansive network of family, friends, and business associates. You may visit her via the web:

Website: https://www.stoneybook.com

Instagram: https://www.instagram.com/bboufford22

NOTES/CREDITS

The song *"Mad World"* by Gary Jules.

https://vallartalifestyles.com/whale-season-2017

http://www.sayulitabeach.com/sayulita-days/

https://barefootsurftravel.com/livemore-magazine/paddle-push-waves

https://www.youtube.com/watch?v=svJk3BR_QTA

The song "Before He Cheats" by Carrie Underwood

https://theculturetrip.com/north-america/mexico/articles/the-reason-why-this-mexican-town-runs-on-a-different-time-zone/

The song "Need You Now" by Lady Antebellum

The song "C'Mon" by Kesha

The song "One" by Metallica

The song "Warriors Of The World United" by Manowar

https://www.twincitieslive.com

https://www.livescience.com/53403-why-sound-of-water-helps-you-sleep.html

https://www.theguardian.com/environment/2013/dec/18/2013-extreme-weather-events

https://en.wikipedia.org/wiki/2013_extreme_weather_events

https://www.ncdc.noaa.gov/sotc/national/201313

NOTES/CREDITS

https://www.youtube.com/watch?v=HBycYHrTCqk YouTube video with channel 12 news
https://www.dw.com/en/why-the-sound-of-waves-is-so-relaxing/av-49386966

https://www.quora.com/Why-is-the-sound-of-waves-crashing-on-a-beach-so-calming

https://www.caringbridge.org/visit/markstoneberg

https://www.startribune.com/riptide-takes-twin-cities-man-out-to-sea-off-mexican-coast/193837551/

https://archive.org/details/Robbinsdale_man_missing_in_Mexico

https://bringmethenews.com/news/search-rescue-professional-joins-effort-to-find-missing-minn-man-in-mexico

https://www.krmg.com/news/local/vacationer-drowns-after-lifeguard-refuses-help/38s33JS3DL1KbD7gUYDDKM/

https://www.news8000.com/body-of-minnesota-man-recovered-in-mexico/

https://patch.com/minnesota/goldenvalley/body-of-missing-robbinsdale-man-found-in-mexico

https://minnesota.cbslocal.com/2013/02/27/mn-man-goes-missing-while-bodysurfing-in-mexico/

https://bringmethenews.com/news/robbinsdale-man-lost-at-sea-after-bodysurfing-in-mexico

https://en.wikipedia.org/wiki/Pacific_Naval_Force

NOTES/CREDITS

https://www.google.com/search?source=hp&ei=F8VqXpXMLcGxtAbS5K
yQAQ&q=miracle+definition&oq=miracle+d&gs_l=psy-
ab.1.0.0i70i249j0l9.2039.8766..12365...3.0..0.92.735.12......0....1..gws-
wiz.......0i131.xSWfX3dFVnU

https://www.hometownsource.com/sun_post/robbinsdale-remember-mark-
stoneberg/article_8d114d46-0226-5cfe-90f9-f9ff2930dfe5.html

https://kstp.com/news/sayulita-mexico-beach-to-honor-robbinsdale-man-
mark-stoneberg-who-drowned-there-with-plaque-at-lifeguard-
tower/4793992/

https://oceanservice.noaa.gov/navigation/tidesandcurrents/

https://oceantoday.noaa.gov/ripcurrentfeature/

http://www.sayulitalife.com/sayulero/index.php/2018/03/01/lifeguard-
tower-dedication-ceremony-in-sayulita/

https://www.ptleader.com/stories/tragedy-in-mexico-zack-died-doing-what-
he-loved,55275

https://www.peninsuladailynews.com/news/emergency-service-fund-set-
up-in-mexico-by-widow-of-port-townsend-man-who-drowned-there/

www.firefighterscrossingborders.org/index.php/regions/region-2-news-
infromation/nayarit

https://www.firefighterscrossingborders.org/index.php/general-news-
informatio/249-sayulita-ifeguard-tower-dedicated

NOTES/CREDITS

https://www.startribune.com/the-story-behind-robbinsdale-s-great-big-sinkhole/216619681/

https://minnesota.cbslocal.com/2013/06/22/sinkhole-opens-up-in-robbinsdale/

https://geospatialresponse.wordpress.com/2013/07/04/recap-twin-cities-severe-weather-event-on-june-21-2013

https://www.ted.com/talks/nora_mcinerny_we_don_t_move_on_from_grief_we_move_forward_with_it?language=en

https://webstore.iec.ch/publication/4150#:~:text=IEC%2061000%2D3%2D3%3A2013%20is%20concerned%20with%20the,guidance%20on%20methods%20of%20assessment

https://www.wunderground.com/history/daily/us/mn/saint-paul/KSTP/date/1999-12-31

https://www.pinterest.com/pin/705657835350660040/memories quote

Scripture quotation marked *NKJV* is taken from the New King James Version of the Bible. Public Domain.

Made in United States
Orlando, FL
10 March 2022

15653104R00143